Fetal alcohol spectrum disorders

A guide for healthcare professionals

June 2007

British Library Cataloguing-in-Publication Data.
A catalogue record for this book is available from the British Library.

ISBN: 1-905545-18-5

Cover photograph: Getty Images Creative

Board of Science

This report was prepared under the auspices of the Board of Science of the British Medical Association, whose membership for 2006/07 was as follows:

Professor Parveen Kumar — President, BMA
Dr Michael Wilks — Chair, BMA Representative Body
Mr James N Johnson — Chair, BMA Council
Dr D Pickersgill — Treasurer, BMA
Sir Charles George — Chair, Board of Science
Dr P B Maguire — Deputy Chair, Board of Science
Dr P H Dangerfield
Dr G D Dilliway
Dr G D Lewis
Dr S Minkoff
Dr O S Moghraby
Dr G Rae
Dr D M Sinclair
Dr A S Thomson
Dr D M B Ward
Dr D G Wrigley
Dr C Spencer-Jones (by invitation)
Dr S Chaudhry (Co-optee)
Dr E F Coyle (Co-optee)
Dr P Miller (Co-optee)
Dr P W Steadman (Co-optee)
Dr S J Nelson (Deputy member)

Approval for publication as a BMA policy report was recommended by BMA Board of Professional Activities on 11 May 2007.

> **Declaration of interest**
> The external reviewers for this report have professional interests in this field. For further information about the editorial secretariat or Board members please contact the Science and Education Department which holds a record of all declarations of interest:
> info.science@bma.org.uk

Acknowledgements

The association is grateful for the help provided by the BMA committees and many outside experts and organisations. We would particularly like to thank:

- Professor Ernest Abel, Professor and Director of Reproductive Toxicology, Department of Obstetrics and Gynecology, C.S. Mott Center, School of Medicine, Wayne State University

- Professor Peter Hepper, Professor of Psychology and Director, Fetal Behaviour Research Centre School of Psychology, Queen's University Belfast & Royal Jubilee Maternity Service

- Dr Raja Mukherjee, Consultant Psychiatrist for People with Learning Disabilities, Surrey and Border Partnership Trust

- Professor Moira Plant, Professor of Alcohol Studies and Co-Director, Alcohol and Health Research Trust, Faculty of Health and Social Care, University of the West of England

- Professor Edward Riley, Professor of Psychology and Director, Center for Behavioural Teratology, San Diego State

Abbreviations

ARBD – alcohol related birth defects
ARND – alcohol related neurodevelopmental disorders
CDC – Centers for Disease Control and Prevention
CKS – clinical knowledge summaries
CNS – central nervous system
CSAT – Centre for Substance Abuse Treatment
DH – Department of Health
DHSS – Department for Health and Social Services
DHSSPS – Department for Health, Social Services and Public Safety
EU – European Union
FASD – fetal alcohol spectrum disorders
FAS – fetal alcohol syndrome
FAST – fast alcohol screening test
FCE – finished consultant episode
GHS – general household survey
GMC – General Medical Council
GP – general practitioner
GUM – genitourinary medicine
HPA – Health Protection Agency
IGF – insulin-like growth factor
IoM – Institute of Medicine
nGMS – new general medical services
NHS – National Health Service
NHSS – national health school standard
NIAAA – National Institute on Alcohol Abuse and Alcoholism
NICE – National Institute for Health and Clinical Excellence
NICHD – National Institute of Child Health and Human Development
NPEU – National Perinatal Epidemiology Unit
NMDA – N-methyl-D-aspartate
ONS – Office for National Statistics
PFAS – partial fetal alcohol syndrome
PMSU – Prime Minister's Strategy Unit
POST – Parliamentary Office of Science and Technology
PSHE – personal, social and health education
RCOG – Royal College of Obstetricians and Gynaecologists
SAMHSA – Substance Abuse and Mental Health Services Administration
SEHD – Scottish Executive Health Department
STI – sexually transmitted infection
SIDS – sudden infant death syndrome
TIPS – treatment improvement protocols
UK – United Kingdom
USA – United States of America

Please note that each time the acronym FASD is used in the text it refers to the full range of disorders that fall within the umbrella term FASD, unless otherwise stated.

Defining alcohol consumption levels

In the UK, alcohol drinks are measured in units and each unit corresponds to 7.9 grams (g) or 10 millilitres (ml) of ethanol. The value of one UK unit does not necessarily correspond to a typical serving size. For example, one unit of alcohol approximates to half a pint of ordinary strength beer, lager, or cider (3–4% alcohol by volume), or a small pub measure (25 ml) of spirits (40% alcohol by volume). There are one and a half units of alcohol in a small glass (125 ml) of ordinary strength wine (12% alcohol by volume), or a standard pub measure (35 ml) of spirits (40% alcohol by volume). There is also considerable variation in the standard measures used in bars and restaurants as well as measures poured in the home. Different methods are used to define standard measurements internationally that may not necessarily correspond to the UK unit.

In studies that report alcohol consumption levels there is little standardisation in the definitions of heavy, moderate and low drinking. For the purposes of this document, low-to-moderate drinking is considered to be less than one drink per day (equivalent to a maximum of 1.5 UK units or 12g of alcohol daily). The Office for National Statistics (ONS) defines heavy drinking as eight or more units for men and six or more units for women on at least one day in the week. Binge drinking can be considered to refer to heavy drinking during the course of an evening or similar time span (ie heavy episodic drinking).[1] Accordingly, the Department of Health (DH) uses the ONS definition of heavy drinking as a proxy for binge drinking. The Prime Minister's Strategy Unit (PMSU) defines binge drinking as drinking over twice the recommended guidelines for daily drinking.

Foreword

Fetal alcohol spectrum disorders (FASD) are a series of completely preventable mental and physical birth defects resulting from maternal alcohol consumption during pregnancy. FASD are lifelong conditions that can significantly impact on the life of the individual and those around them as illustrated by the case studies included within this report.

This report focuses on the adverse health impacts of alcohol consumption during pregnancy, and in particular the problem of FASD. It continues the work of the Board on alcohol and public health which has resulted in a number of publications including *Binge drinking* (2005), *Adolescent health* (2003), *Alcohol and young people* (1999), *Alcohol: guidelines on sensible drinking* (1995), and *The BMA guide to alcohol and accidents* (1989).

The report aims to raise awareness of FASD by examining the incidence, cause and outcomes of the range of disorders associated with alcohol consumption during pregnancy. It further outlines the responsibilities of healthcare professionals and the wider medical community in managing and reducing the incidence of these disorders. This report is intended for healthcare professionals and relevant bodies with strategic or operational responsibility for public health and health promotion.

[signature]

Professor Sir Charles George
Chair, Board of Science

> The Board of Science, a standing committee of the BMA, provides an interface between the medical profession, the government and the public. The Board produces numerous reports containing policies for national action by government and other organisations, with specific recommendations affecting the medical and allied professions.

Contents

Introduction

Alcohol is a teratogenic compound (ie a substance which interferes with the normal development of the embryo or fetus) that readily crosses the placenta. In the absence of a developed blood filtration system, the fetus is totally unprotected from alcohol circulating in the blood system. Prenatal alcohol exposure can affect the fetus in a number of ways. The most devastating effects are the intellectual disabilities associated with the adverse impact of alcohol on fetal brain development and the central nervous system (CNS). Damage to the brain is often, though not always, accompanied by distinctive facial deformities, physical and emotional developmental problems, memory and attention deficits, and a variety of cognitive and behavioural problems. Further complications such as mental illness and alcohol and drug addiction may also develop. Over the past 30 years, considerable attention has focused on the role of prenatal alcohol exposure in the occurrence of a wide range of disorders classified under the umbrella term FASD. These disorders range in diversity from the full presentation of Fetal Alcohol Syndrome (FAS), to a set of conditions – including Partial Fetal Alcohol Syndrome (PFAS),[a] Alcohol-Related Birth Defects (ARBD) and Alcohol-Related Neurodevelopmental Disorders (ARND) – that show some, but not all of the features of FAS.[2] The extra cost of FASD has been estimated in the United States of America (USA) at $500,000 per individual over a 20-year period.[2] The adjusted lifetime cost for each individual with FAS has been estimated at US$2 million.[3]

Although a significant amount of research has focused on FASD, particularly in Canada and the USA, there has been limited work on this in the United Kingdom (UK). Determining the incidence of FASD is complicated by a lack of reliable and consistent data collection, and the difficulty in diagnosing the range of disorders. Consequently, the incidence of FASD in the UK and internationally is not accurately known. The relationship between maternal alcohol consumption and the development of the range of disorders is not fully understood. The level and pattern of alcohol consumption, and the stage of pregnancy during which alcohol is consumed are important determinants of the outcome of an alcohol-affected pregnancy.[4, 5]

FASD are completely preventable through the elimination of drinking during pregnancy. In the UK, recent years have seen a significant rise in the number of women of childbearing age who drink heavily.[6, 7, 8] Prevention requires a good understanding of the continuum of permanent birth defects associated with FASD and an increased awareness of the risks of prenatal alcohol exposure among the general public, and in particular women who are pregnant or considering a pregnancy. There is, however, evidence suggesting that FASD are a set of conditions that is poorly understood in the UK by the general public and healthcare professionals.[2] Further preventative measures include screening of pregnant women for maternal alcohol consumption, referral for brief interventions, and targeting of women at high risk of an alcohol-affected pregnancy. The management of FASD necessitates cooperation between a wide range of healthcare professionals as well as individuals in the fields of education and social services.[2] Following diagnosis it is vital that appropriate treatment and support systems are implemented at the earliest possible stage to prevent the onset of secondary problems.

---

[a] PFAS is also termed Possible Fetal Alcohol Effects (PFAE).

Fetal alcohol spectrum disorders

The adverse effects of prenatal alcohol exposure on the developing fetus and child lie within a continuum and represent a spectrum of structural anomalies, and behavioural and neurocognitive impairments. The range of phenotypes associated with FASD vary in severity and clinical outcome depending on the level, pattern, and timing of maternal alcohol consumption. Individuals defined as having FAS – which is the most clinically recognisable form of FASD – exhibit the full phenotype which is characterised by a pattern of anomalies including:

- CNS dysfunction – damage to the CNS results in the permanent impairment of brain function that may lead to intellectual and developmental disabilities, attention deficits, poor social understanding, hyperactivity, learning disabilities, poor coordination and planning, poor muscle tone, working memory deficits, receptive language deficits, executive functioning deficits (eg difficulty in organising and planning), and the inability to learn from the consequences of their behaviour
- facial dysmorphology – FAS is commonly associated with abnormal facial features including short palpebral fissures, a thin upper lip vermillion and a smooth philtrum
- pre- and post-natal growth deficiency – babies born with FAS are commonly smaller than other babies and typically remain smaller throughout their lives.[9]

The clinical features of PFAS, ARBD and ARND are less well defined. With each phenotype, the affected individuals exhibit some, but not all, of the characteristic triad of anomalies associated with FAS (as above). PFAS, ARBD and ARND are not necessarily less severe than FAS, however, as the individual anomalies associated with these conditions may confer the same level of damage that occurs in FAS. Children affected by PFAS usually display a characteristic pattern of minor facial anomalies, deficits encompassing intellectual disabilities, hyperactivity with attention deficit, impulsivity, short attention span, and are developmentally delayed in comparison to other children.[10] ARND are characterised by the presence of prominent neurocognitive deficits and the absence of growth and facial anomalies. Children with ARBD have pronounced behavioural features or congenital structural abnormalities, but lack most of the facial anomalies characteristic of FAS. For illustrations of the characteristics associated with FASD see appendix 1.

The neurocognitive deficits associated with CNS dysfunction mean that individuals affected by FASD may experience additional problems as a result of difficulties in learning, judgement, planning and memory. These include psychiatric problems, disrupted school experience, trouble with the law, confinement, alcohol and drug problems, and inappropriate sexual behaviour.[2]

Epidemiology

There is currently no reliable evidence on the incidence of FASD in the UK. In England and Scotland, data are only collected on FAS and not the whole spectrum of FASD. According to the DH Hospital Episode Statistics, the number of cases of FAS in England was 95 in 2000-01, 90 in 2001-02 and 128 in 2002-03.[11] In Scotland, there were four cases of FAS in 2000, five in 2001, four in 2002, two in 2003 and 10 cases in 2004.[12] This equated to 0.21 per 1,000 live births in 2004.[12] There are currently no data available for the incidence of FAS in Northern Ireland or Wales. In the USA, the incidence of FAS is reported to be between 0.5 and 2 per 1,000 live births.[13] The reported worldwide incidence of FAS is 0.97 cases per 1,000.[14] It is important to note, however, that this estimate is based almost entirely on data from the USA.[14] FAS, although not a common condition, is nevertheless regarded as the leading known cause of non-genetic intellectual disability in the Western world.[15]

Data on the incidence of the full range of FASD are continuing to emerge and it is clear that some populations are more likely to have children affected by these disorders. The most at risk populations are those that experience high degrees of social deprivation and poverty such as indigenous or native populations. In Australian aboriginal populations the incidence of FASD is estimated as 4.7 per 1,000 live births,[16] while the incidence in the Western Cape Province of South Africa has been reported to be as high as 68.0 to 89.2 per 1,000 children.[17] The incidence of FASD in Italy has been estimated to be 20.3 to 40.5 per 1,000 children.[18] In Canada, FASD are reported to affect 10 in every 1,000 live births.[19] It has been estimated that in Western countries as many as 9 per 1,000 live births involve children affected by FAS, PFAS or ARND.[20] Of the children concerned, 10 to 15 per cent are affected by FAS, 30 to 40 per cent by PFAS, and nearly half by ARND.[20]

A key complication in determining the incidence of FASD is the absence of robust and routine data collection in the UK and internationally. This is partly due to the current uncertainty and debate regarding the range of conditions associated with prenatal alcohol exposure and the difficulty in the diagnosis of the range of FASD (see section on diagnosis and referral). In 2005 the Centers for Disease Control and Prevention (CDC) noted that FAS is currently the only diagnostic category with scientific evidence to support clinical criteria.[21] It is worth noting that, worryingly, FAS is a disorder, the existence of which is still debated in the UK. This may explain why data on FASD are not routinely collected in the UK, and, where data are collected, are restricted to FAS. In some countries including Australia, Canada, New Zealand and the USA, FAS is or has been one of the diagnostic categories for which data are collected by the respective National Paediatric Surveillance Units. These data are not currently recorded by the British Paediatric Surveillance Unit (BPSU).[b] It is essential that data on FAS are routinely collected throughout the UK and consideration is given to how this should be extended to the full range of FASD. Further research is required to determine the incidence and prevalence of FASD in the UK and internationally.

Recommendations
- The UK health departments should ensure data on FAS are routinely collected throughout the UK and consider how this should be extended to cover the range of FASD.
- Further research should be undertaken to establish the epidemiology of the range of FASD in the UK through an increased recognition of these disorders, improved data collection and UK-based research. This should build on existing data and highlight the differences in populations through coordinated large-scale national and international studies.

---

[b] The BPSU, which is currently funded by the DH, undertakes active surveillance of rare conditions in children in the UK and the Republic of Ireland.

Neilette's story...

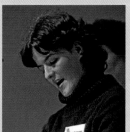 My name is Neilette. I am 20 years old. Because I have FAS people stare at me. It makes me feel angry. I say to them what are you staring at and they just walk away.

My mum was 40 when I was born. Mum and Dad found out I had FAS when I was born. They didn't tell me straight away. They told me I had FAS when I was about nine. My Mum also died when I was about nine.

When I was younger, I got the 'mickey' taken out of me from all the kids on the street. I got used to it. Kids bullied me in school and I had a fight and broke my ankle.

Then I went to a special boarding school in Gloucester when I was 11 until I was 14. It was terrible. I hated it. I ran away and took the train to London and went to Dad.

They took me back to boarding school but I only stayed for a week. Then I moved back to London to a special unit in Becton for people with special needs. I was there for two years. There was 12 of us. It was alright.

I lived with Tasha who was a self-harmer. After two years the term was over and I had to leave and I moved back with my Dad.

It's hard for me to handle money and make change, but I do pay half my bills. It's also hard for me to remember things. If my Dad asks me to go down to the shops to get four things I come back with three things because it is difficult to remember. It's hard for me to keep friends.

The good things in my life are my Dad and the MAP Newspaper. It's a paper for people with learning disabilities. I am the advertising manager. I go in every day. I made some nice friends. The fire brigade man wants to put some advertising in the paper. And that's all down to me.

Another good thing is my dog, Sophie. She's an Alsatian Collie.

I think my life is difficult because I am not the same as anyone else and that makes my life difficult. The things that are difficult are like having friends and knowing they are not really your friends.

I wish people were more understanding.

What I think people should know about FAS, they should come to [National Organisation on Fetal Alcohol Syndrome] NOFAS and learn about it.

Alcohol consumption in women of childbearing age and during pregnancy

Approximately 90 per cent of women in Britain consume alcoholic beverages at least occasionally,[22, 23, 24] and there has recently been a significant increase in heavy drinking among young British women.[6, 7, 8] A survey in 2000 showed that eight per cent of women aged 18-24 years had consumed at least 35 units of alcohol during the previous week.[25, 26] A study of drinking trends in the UK found 38 per cent of women in their 20s had engaged in binge drinking.[6] The General Household Survey (GHS) 2003 found that the proportion of women aged 16-24 years who had consumed six units or more on at least one day in the past week had risen from 24 per cent to 28 per cent over the period 1998-2002.[27] It also found that women aged 16-24 were far more likely than other age groups to have consumed six units or more in one day and that nine per cent of all women aged 16 and above were heavy drinkers in 2003. A report from the Parliamentary Office of Science and Technology (POST) found that 60 per cent of alcohol consumed by women aged 20 to 29 is consumed in bouts of heavy drinking.[28]

The increasing level of alcohol consumption among women in the UK has been accompanied by a substantial rise in alcohol-related morbidity and mortality. According to the ONS, the number of alcohol-related deaths among UK women aged 35-54 years has doubled between 1991 and 2005, from 7.2 to 14.2 per 100,000 population.[29] Recent years have seen a significant rise in deaths from liver disease in England and Wales and an increasing proportion of such deaths involve relatively young adults.[30] In 2000, cirrhosis accounted for nearly 300 deaths in women aged 25-44 years. In the past decade the most common age for mortality from chronic liver disease has dropped from 55-64 years to 45-54 years.[30] If the age at which the onset of chronic liver disease continues to fall this may increasingly affect women of childbearing age who may be at risk of becoming pregnant with a liver which is already less able to process alcohol efficiently.

In the 2000 UK survey on infant feeding,[c] the reported rates of drinking during pregnancy were found to have declined consistently since 1995 when two-thirds of mothers throughout the UK consumed alcohol during pregnancy.[31] The survey found that 87 per cent of mothers had sometimes consumed alcohol before pregnancy; around six in 10 drank alcohol while they were pregnant, and approximately three in 10 drinkers gave up during pregnancy.[31] In 2000, 71 per cent of a sample of mothers who continued to drink during their pregnancy reported drinking on average less than one unit of alcohol in a week.[31] In light of the recent increasing levels of alcohol consumption in women of childbearing age in the UK, it is reasonable to suggest that this will lead to an increased risk of heavy drinking during pregnancy and subsequently an increased risk of having a baby who is effected by pre-natal alcohol exposure.

According to the 2003 BMA report, *Adolescent health*, adolescents in the UK have one of the highest levels of alcohol use, binge-drinking and getting drunk in Europe.[32] The rate of teenage pregnancies in the UK is the highest in Western Europe.[33] In England and Wales the rate of conception in women under 18 was 41.3 per 1,000 in 2005,[34] and in Scotland it was 42.4 per 1,000 in 2003-04.[35] In Northern Ireland, 6.9 per cent of total live births in 2001 were to women under the age of 20.[36] The rate of sexually transmitted infections (STIs) in the UK increased significantly between 1996 and 2005 with the numbers of individuals presenting with an STI at genitourinary medicine (GUM) clinics across the UK increasing by 60 per cent.[37] Recent evidence suggests that unplanned pregnancies are common,[38, 39] not only in young women but in women throughout their childbearing years.[40] Many women will not therefore know they are pregnant during the early part of the first trimester, during which time they may continue to drink in their pre-pregnancy fashion with no awareness of the risk to their unborn child.

---

c This survey was conducted jointly on behalf of the DH, the Scottish Executive Health Department (SEHD), the National Assembly for Wales and the Department of Health, Social Services and Public Safety (DHSSPS) in Northern Ireland.

Underestimating maternal alcohol consumption

Data on rates of drinking during pregnancy are commonly based on self reporting and therefore often unreliable as a result of poor estimation, poor recollection and the social stigma associated with heavy drinking during pregnancy. This is compounded by variation in the alcoholic concentration of different types of drink, variation in serving size (ie different sizes of wine glass), and the difference between the standard measures used in bars and restaurants as well as measures poured in the home. Maternal alcohol consumption levels are therefore often significantly underestimated.[4] This can lead to difficulties in studying the association between alcohol and poor health outcome, and in recording patient histories of alcohol consumption. Underestimating alcohol consumption can also affect an individual's perceptions of their level of drinking and how much they think is safe to drink.

Is there a safe level of exposure to alcohol during pregnancy?

The damage caused by alcohol on the developing fetus is dependent on the level of maternal alcohol consumption, the pattern of alcohol exposure and the stage of pregnancy during which alcohol is consumed.[41] This is confounded by a number of other risk factors including the genetic makeup of the mother and the fetus, the nutritional status of the mother, hormonal interactions, polydrug use (including tobacco use), general health of the mother, stress, maternal age and low socioeconomic status.[2, 42-44] For example, research to identify specific genetic factors contributing to FASD has found that polymorphisms of the gene for the alcohol dehydrogenase enzyme ADH1B in both the mother and the fetus, can contribute to FASD vulnerability.[45]

There is robust and consistent evidence from human and animal studies that heavy maternal alcohol use is associated with FAS.[4, 5] This is particularly apparent in cases of alcohol dependence or severe alcohol problems;[5] however, only four to five per cent of children born to women who consumed large amounts of alcohol during pregnancy are affected by the full syndrome presentation.[4] The pattern and duration of drinking are important considerations in defining the risk of heavy drinking during pregnancy. The occurrence of FAS has been found to be associated with the frequency of heavy dose drinking (ie binge drinking).[14] Women who binge drink are much more likely to have children with facial dysmorphology, cardiac anomalies or cognitive impairment than women who drink the same total amount of alcohol over an extended period of time.[43]

The stage of pregnancy during which alcohol is consumed determines how and which cells of the developing fetus are affected. Research has shown there to be vulnerable periods of neonatal development that can be adversely affected by exposure to heavy doses of alcohol intake.[2, 4, 5, 41] Evidence from animal experiments suggests these critical periods of exposure occur during the first and third trimesters in humans. Studies in mice have found the very early stages of embryogenesis to be critical periods for damage to the developing brain and induction of alcohol-induced craniofacial alterations.[46-49] Prenatal alcohol exposure during the third trimester is highly-related to damage to the cerebellum, hippocampus and prefrontal cortex.[41] A small-scale study examining children with school problems who had been prenatally exposed to alcohol found that damage to the cerebellum can also occur following heavy maternal alcohol consumption during the first trimester of pregnancy.[50] The occurrence of PFAS, ARBD and ARND is not fully understood. It has been postulated that the anomalies characteristic of PFAS, ARBD and ARND result from exposure to heavy doses of alcohol intake on specific days of fetal development, and that exposure to heavy doses throughout pregnancy results in the development of the pattern of anomalies found in FAS.[43]

There is considerable debate as to the adverse effects of maternal alcohol consumption at low-to-moderate levels of drinking. This may be explained by the variability in the definitions of consumption levels, differences in the way drinking behaviour is characterised, methodological problems in the design and analysis of relevant studies, and in determining the relative effect of confounding factors (eg genetic predisposition).

Existing evidence on the adverse irreversible effects of prenatal alcohol exposure at low-to-moderate levels is inconclusive and there is currently no consensus on the level of risk or whether there is a clear threshold below which alcohol is non-teratogenic. A 2006 review of the existing evidence on the effects of alcohol on the developing embryo, fetus and child conducted by the National Perinatal Epidemiology Unit (NPEU) found there to be no consistent evidence of adverse health effects from low-to-moderate prenatal alcohol exposure.[4] Other reviews have drawn similar conclusions.[44, 51] It is worth noting that the current evidence is not robust enough to exclude any risk from low-to-moderate levels,[4] and that evidence is continuing to emerge as to the possible effects of prenatal alcohol exposure at these levels. Evidence from animal experiments suggests that damage to the CNS may occur at low levels of alcohol exposure.[2, 4, 52, 53] Moreover, a prospective study of 501 mother-child dyads found that the child's behaviour at age six to seven was adversely related to low-to-moderate levels of prenatal alcohol exposure.[54] A dose-response relationship between the level of alcohol consumed and the behaviour exhibited was also found.[54] Studies examining the effects of alcohol on the fetus have shown that exposure at low-to-moderate levels can alter fetal behaviour (see appendix 2). These studies have consistently shown that acute exposure to one to two units of alcohol rapidly suppresses fetal behaviour through a rapid decrease in fetal breathing.[55-58] Studies examining the effects of chronic consumption indicate that low-to-moderate levels of exposure (two to five units per week) elicit a developmental delay in the functioning of the fetus's nervous system and may result in a permanent effect.[59, 60] It is not currently clear what effect these changes in behaviour have on fetal development and the health outcomes of pregnancy. A recent large prospective study has found that occasional low-to-moderate drinking during the first trimester may have a negative and persistent effect on children's mental health.[61]

Clarification is required as to the effect of different levels, patterns and timings of prenatal alcohol exposure on the health outcomes of pregnancy. There is a significant amount of research currently focused on this area. It is important that this is consolidated with further research to generate a consensus on the relationship between different levels of prenatal alcohol exposure and the range of conditions associated with FASD. This should then help inform the debate on whether there is a safe threshold for prenatal alcohol exposure. As many of the epidemiological methods used to examine the risk factors associated with FASD rely on retrospective extrapolation from existing cases and information, it is important that future research – if methodologically possible – is based on a prospective ascertainment process of whole populations with better recording and stratification of alcohol dose levels.

Recommendation
- Further research should be undertaken in the UK to examine the relationship between prenatal alcohol exposure and the range of conditions associated with FASD. This research should build on existing work in this area and occur via population screening that is based on an active ascertainment process.

Maternal alcohol consumption – effects on the fetus

Prenatal alcohol exposure is likely to exert its effects via two broad mechanisms. Firstly, ethanol is a teratogenic compound that readily crosses the placenta. Evidence from animal studies has found that the disruption of normal fetal developmental processes is likely to occur via multiple mechanisms.[2, 4, 5, 62, 63] The various potential mechanisms of alcohol teratogenesis can be grouped into the categories as in box 1.

Box 1 – potential mechanisms of ethanol teratogenesis

- *Disruption of cellular energetics* – altered glucose utilization and transport, suppression of protein and DNA synthesis, oxidative stress
- *Impairment of cell acquisition/dysregulation of developmental timing* – altered cell cycle, impaired neurogenesis and gliogenesis, mistimed events of cell generation, migration, neurite outgrowth, synaptogenesis, and myelination
- *Altered regulation of gene expression* – reduced retinoic acid signalling, effects on other transcription factors
- *Disrupted cell-cell interactions* – inhibition of L1 cell adhesion molecule (L1 CAM) function
- *Interference with growth factor signalling or other cell-signalling pathways* – reduced functioning of N-methyl-D-aspartate (NMDA) receptors, delayed development of the serotonin system, inhibition of insulin-like growth factors (IGF) I and II
- *Cell damage/cell death* – apoptosis, oxidative stress, withdrawal-induced glutamatergic excitotoxicity
- *Secondary sources of damage* – altered placental function or other intrauterine factors, hypoxia/ischaemia, acetaldehyde formation.[5, 62, 63]

These mechanisms are most likely activated at different stages of fetal development and may contribute to the varying patterns of anomalies associated with the various FASD phenotypes.[63] It is important to note that none of the mechanisms can account for all of the different anomalies individually and there is likely to be significant overlap between the mechanism pathways.[62] The resultant premature cell death and disruption of the normal development and placement of cells significantly impacts on fetal development. While this can cause abnormalities in the physical structure of the fetus and impair fetal growth, the impact on neural development is the most debilitating feature of prenatal alcohol exposure. Cells in the CNS experience more rapid cell death than other cells in the developing embryo as they have a lower toxicity threshold for alcohol.[5] Prenatal alcohol exposure also causes widespread damage to the CNS by disrupting normal neural developmental process (eg maturation of glial cells).[5] This primarily affects the areas of the brain – including the basal ganglia, the corpus callosum, the cerebellum, and, to some degree, the hippocampus – that are responsible for motor and cognitive skills, learning, memory, and executive functioning,[5] all of which may be impaired in FAS.

A second mechanism of action may be the persistent changes in fetal behaviour resulting from alcohol exposure. It is now recognised that prenatal development is not just under genetic control but that the fetus's sensory environment, and motor behaviour actions and reactions all contribute to the normal developmental process.[64] Maternal alcohol consumption has the potential to cause permanent damage to the fetus through continual disruption of the normal developmental processes (see appendix 2). The effects of continual disruption of these processes are unknown. It is important that further research is undertaken to clarify the exact mechanisms of ethanol teratogenesis and establish how they relate to the pattern of anomalies associated with FASD.

Recommendation
- Further research should be undertaken to clarify the exact mechanisms of ethanol teratogenesis and establish how they relate to the pattern of anomalies associated with FASD.

Other adverse health outcomes of maternal alcohol consumption

The effects of maternal alcohol consumption are not limited to the range of FASD. Alcohol can adversely impact on the reproductive process in a number of ways, including:

- infertility – heavy drinking and chronic alcohol misuse is associated with an increased risk of infertility and higher rates of menstrual disorders.[51, 65] Alcohol consumption by women is also associated with a decreased chance of becoming pregnant [65]
- miscarriage – alcohol consumption is associated with an increased risk of miscarriage as a result of the development of aneuploidy or major structural malformations of the fetus [51]
- pre-term deliveries and stillbirth – high levels of maternal alcohol consumption in early and late pregnancy is associated with pre-term labour,[51] and low-to-moderate levels of consumption are associated with an increased risk of stillbirth.[66] Research conducted by the National Institute of Child Health and Human Development (NICHD) and the National Institute on Alcohol Abuse and Alcoholism (NIAAA) has found that prenatal alcohol exposure may be associated with an increased risk of sudden infant death syndrome (SIDS).[67]

Susan's story...

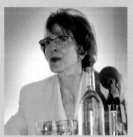

The first time I heard about FAS I was sitting in a medical lecture. When the speaker discussed the eight main characteristics of FAS, my 10-year-old daughter had seven of them. When he said children with FAS have a 'smaller than normal head circumference', bells went off. I had been to six bicycle shops and no one had a children's bicycle helmet small enough for my daughter's head.

Within weeks I had a confirmed diagnosis at Great Ormond Street Hospital... my adopted daughter had FAS. I knew her birth mother was an alcoholic, but never knew that would affect my child for the rest of her life. Now, nine years later, I can recognise many children like my daughter. She is part of a universal family of children prenatally damaged by alcohol.

Because of her mature vocabulary and witty sense of humour people presume my daughter is a very bright 19 year old. Though the parts of her brain that weren't damaged by alcohol are very clever, in reality, she has an IQ of 75 and the maturity of someone half her age.

What she can do today, she may not be able to do tomorrow. She gets angry at herself and hits herself. Her legs are black and blue. Others get angry at her when she is not consistent. When I tried to explain this to a teacher, I was told, I know your daughter can do it, she did it before, she's just not trying.

Like the majority of people with FAS, my daughter can't tell time, do maths or give change. At age 19 her peers have outgrown her. Her closest friend is 12. She is isolated and depressed and often talks about suicide. I love her dearly and I feel her pain.

Children with FAS get punished for their disability. Because they look normal, they are punished for being lazy, stubborn and defiant. The reality is, they can't remember, they can't understand and they can't explain. Some say living with FAS is like having to find one's way around Liverpool with a map of Glasgow.

I know many families whose children got the diagnosis too late. Their children have been excluded from school, have run away, become homeless, been victims of violence and abuse, are in prison or have committed suicide.

My daughter is lucky because, by chance, I learned about FAS. Though her life will never be normal, it is always improving. She recently took third place in the Riding for the Disabled, RDA Nationals.

When parents, schools, doctors and social services know what they are dealing with we can begin to improve lives for children like my daughter and everyone affected. My daughter's disability could have been prevented. Her life is my greatest lesson.

Susan Fleisher,
Founder of NOFAS-UK (National Organisation for Fetal Alcohol Syndrome-UK) and the FASD Medical Advisory Panel, the NOFAS-UK Family Support Network. www.nofas-uk.org

Awareness of fetal alcohol spectrum disorders in the medical profession

The prevention and management of the continuum of FASD necessitates a good understanding of these disorders among healthcare professionals, including their relationship with maternal alcohol consumption, what intervention strategies are effective, and how they are diagnosed and managed. There is, however, anecdotal evidence from unpublished data and national, regional and local conferences that FASD are a set of conditions that is poorly understood by healthcare professionals in the UK.[2, 68] This is in part due to a lack of consensus in the scientific literature regarding FASD. The lack of understanding among healthcare professionals in the UK is reflected internationally.[69-73] In the USA, a survey of paediatricians found that even though they were knowledgeable about FAS, they did not feel adequately trained to integrate the management, diagnosis or prevention methods into everyday practice, and were not active in routine anticipatory guidance with adolescents for prevention of alcohol-affected pregnancies.[70] Research is needed in order to examine the current levels of understanding and knowledge of FASD by healthcare professionals in the UK. A lack of knowledge about FASD will limit opportunities for diagnosis, prevention and early intervention. It is therefore important that efforts are made to provide training and guidance, and increase awareness of FASD among healthcare professionals.

Recommendations
- Research should be undertaken to determine the current levels of understanding and knowledge of the range of FASD among healthcare professionals in the UK.
- The UK health departments should implement training programmes for healthcare professionals on the prevention, diagnosis and management of the range of FASD.

Prevention of fetal alcohol spectrum disorders

The prevention of FASD requires a coordinated and multi-faceted approach that incorporates universal prevention strategies aimed at the general population (eg public awareness and educational campaigns), selective prevention strategies aimed at women of childbearing age, in particular those who are considering a pregnancy (eg screening for maternal alcohol consumption), and specific prevention strategies aimed at women who are at high-risk (eg referral to specialist alcohol services).

Sensible drinking guidelines

There is clear evidence that heavy drinking adversely impacts on the developing fetus; yet, as discussed earlier it is unclear whether there is any safe level of maternal alcohol consumption.[4, 5, 9, 44, 51] This has led to variation in the guidelines in the UK on alcohol consumption during pregnancy (see appendix 3). There is no conclusive evidence that drinking at the maximum levels recommended in current UK guidance – approximately one to two units per week – is harmful to the developing fetus.[4, 44, 51] Evidence is continuing to emerge however as to the possible risks of prenatal alcohol exposure at low-to-moderate levels.[53, 54, 59-61] It is also important to note that guidelines on sensible drinking can be misinterpreted as individuals may not clearly understand what units or 'standard drinks' are.[8] This could lead to confusion about what sensible drinking really is.[8] Given the current uncertainty regarding the level of risk to the developing fetus, and the lack of clear guidelines, the only safe sensible drinking message is not to drink any alcohol during pregnancy. As previously noted, unplanned pregnancies are common and many women of childbearing age in the UK engage in episodic heavy or binge drinking. It is therefore crucial that women considering a pregnancy are aware of the risks associated with alcohol consumption during pregnancy. In the USA, the US Surgeon General recommends that women who are pregnant or who may become pregnant should abstain from consuming alcohol.[74]

Recommendations
- Women who are pregnant, or who are considering a pregnancy, should be advised not to consume any alcohol.
- The UK health departments should work in partnership with relevant stakeholder organisations to revise current guidance on sensible drinking (see appendix 3). They should ensure that consistent and clear advice is given to healthcare professionals and the general public regarding the sensible drinking message and the risks of alcohol consumption during pregnancy.

Universal prevention strategies

Universal prevention strategies are aimed at the entire population (national, local community, school, neighbourhood). While their effects are often limited at this level, they can be useful in changing attitudes among particular groups. Universal strategies for preventing FASD include the implementation of effective public health policies that raise awareness of the risks of maternal alcohol consumption and alter drinking behaviour, both prior to conception and during pregnancy.

In the USA, a number of specific universal strategies aimed at preventing FASD have been used. These have focused on media advertising campaigns, school and community-based programmes, warning posters, and labelling of alcohol beverages.[d] With the exception of alcohol beverage warning labels, there has been relatively little research into the effectiveness of universal FASD prevention strategies in the USA.[75] A number of small surveys found the use of warning posters produced a modest increase in awareness regarding the adverse effects of alcohol consumption during pregnancy.[75] Analysis of the impact of alcohol beverage warning labels found there to be an increase in awareness and knowledge

---

[d] Alcohol beverage warning labels were introduced in the USA in 1989 following implementation of the Alcoholic Beverage Warning Label Act 1988.

of FASD among the general public, and in particular, in young women.[5, 9, 75-77] The labelling was found to have only modest effects on personal risk perceptions and drinking behaviours.[9, 75, 76] A modest reduction in alcohol consumption during pregnancy was seen eight months after the introduction of the warning label;[e] however, this decrease was short-lived and alcohol consumption levels had returned to normal by 1995.[9, 75, 78] This transitory reduction occurred only in women who were light drinkers and there was no significant change among those drinking at risk levels.[9] Therefore, despite the increase in awareness of the range of FASD, the introduction of warning labels did not result in long-term decreases in alcohol consumption.

In the UK, there have been no universal strategies focused specifically on preventing these disorders. It is unclear whether this is because FASD are perceived to be a minor problem, or because it is felt such strategies are ineffective. The current UK strategy for reducing alcohol-related harm focuses on health promotion through effective communication of the sensible drinking message; school-based educational programmes; responsible advertising and service policies; and enforcement of licensing laws (see appendix 4). Research examining these types of alcohol control policy has shown them to be largely ineffective. Reviews of the efficacy of alcohol education and health promotion have consistently concluded that they are not effective measures for altering drinking behaviour or reducing alcohol-related harm in a population.[8, 79] School-based educational programmes have been found to increase knowledge and modify attitudes; yet they have been shown to have limited effect on drinking behaviour in the long-term.[8, 79] Only a small number of credible educational programmes have been found to reduce young people's drinking.[8] Controlling the price and availability of alcoholic drinks has been shown to be effective at reducing alcohol-related problems and population mean alcohol consumption level.[4, 79] These measures could potentially be effective in reducing alcohol consumption during pregnancy. These policies, however, have proved unpopular politically in the UK, and have not been used as part of the strategy to reduce alcohol-related harm.

The introduction of public health policies aimed at preventing the range of FASD need to be considered within the context of the overall alcohol-related harm strategy. Universal strategies to prevent FASD by reducing levels of alcohol consumption during pregnancy need to include policies that alter drinking behaviour and reduce population mean alcohol consumption. This necessitates the introduction of evidence-based policies that decrease the affordability of alcohol and limit its availability. A Private Members' Bill proposing the introduction of the warning labels on alcoholic products in the UK has recently had a second reading in the House of Lords and is awaiting the Committee stage.[f] In England, the DH is currently reviewing the 2004 alcohol harm-reduction strategy and is expected to outline a new strategy in 2007. In February 2007, the Scottish Executive Published *Plan for action on alcohol problems: update* which provides an update on the original 2002 strategy and refers to plans to work with the UK government (and the drinks industry) to discuss labelling.[80] While health promotion and educational programmes may have a role in modifying attitudes and raising awareness of the risks of alcohol consumption during pregnancy, they have not been shown to have any significant effect on drinking behaviour.[8, 79] It is therefore essential that such measures are used to support other policies that are effective at altering drinking behaviour. For example, combining public education and price increases has been found to be particularly effective in reducing alcohol consumption in women who drink heavily.[81]

---

[e] This reduction was found in a study of 21,127 pregnant African American women using an inner-city prenatal clinic between 1986 and 1995.

[f] The Alcohol Labelling Bill was introduced to the House of Lords by Lord Mitchell. The first reading of the Bill was on 29 January 2007, and the second reading was on 20 April 2007.

Further research is required to identify the most effective measures to raise awareness of the full range of FASD and prevent alcohol consumption during pregnancy in the UK. This in turn requires an understanding of current attitudes and levels of awareness relating to alcohol consumption during pregnancy and FASD. In light of the high level of adolescent drinking and teenage pregnancy in the UK, there is also an urgent need to establish the most effective measures to raise awareness among this age group.

Recommendations

- The UK government should review existing alcohol control policies in the UK to ensure that they are evidence-based and effective. This should include the introduction of increased taxation on alcohol products and the implementation of policies limiting the availability of alcohol. Any changes to existing alcohol control policies should be regularly reviewed and evaluated.
- Health promotion, and public and school-based educational programmes aimed at preventing FASD should only be used as part of a wider alcohol-related harm reduction strategy to support other policies that are effective at altering drinking behaviour.
- Research should be undertaken to establish current public attitudes and levels of awareness of FASD in the UK and the risks of alcohol consumption during pregnancy among the general public.
- Further research should be undertaken to identify the most effective ways to educate the public about the range of FASD and to alter drinking behaviour. This requires systematic studies that compare various universal prevention strategies and their impacts across the different social groups.

Selective and indicated prevention – the role of the healthcare professional

Healthcare professionals are well placed to implement selective and indicated prevention strategies. Selective prevention strategies target all women of childbearing age and include health promotion and advice, screening of pregnant women for alcohol use, and the implementation of brief interventions as appropriate. Indicated prevention strategies are targeted at women who are at high-risk of having children affected by FASD and includes treatment of alcohol addiction problems where present.

Health promotion and advice
Healthcare professionals have a specific responsibility in providing advice to their patients – both prior to conception and during pregnancy – on the risks associated with maternal alcohol consumption and on sensible drinking guidelines. This is in addition to the advice provided to patients on other lifestyle choices such as smoking habits and nutrition. In the 2000 UK infant feeding survey, 77 per cent of pregnant women reported being given some information about alcohol consumption during pregnancy, which was substantially more than the six per cent reported in 1995.[31] Advice was most commonly provided by a midwife (83%) and just under a third received advice from a doctor (31%, down from 41% in 1995).[31]

As part of routine clinical care, general practitioners (GPs) have a responsibility to provide information and advice on FASD prevention to women who are considering a pregnancy, as appropriate, and to record their history of alcohol use. In the antenatal setting, GPs, obstetricians and members of the wider healthcare team (eg midwives) have a responsibility to provide ongoing advice and support to expectant mothers at every stage of pregnancy and this should include information on the risks of maternal alcohol consumption.[9] It is essential that the advice provided by healthcare professionals is up to date, consistent and evidence-based. This health advice should be supplemented with 'take home' printed information. The combination of verbal guidance together with printed information has been found to decrease alcohol consumption levels in pregnant women.[10] The sources of further information section at the end of this report lists details of patient information resources.

Recommendations
- All healthcare professionals as a part of routine clinical care should provide ongoing advice and support to expectant mothers at every stage of pregnancy and this should include information on the risks of maternal alcohol consumption.
- All health promotion and advice should be supplemented with 'take home' printed information on the risks of consuming alcohol during pregnancy.
  Printed information should be:
  - clear and concise
  - available for all healthcare professionals and primary care organisations to use
  - reviewed to ensure that they are targeted at the population at risk including difficult to reach groups.

Monitoring and detecting maternal alcohol consumption
Effective prevention of the range of FASD requires the accurate identification of pregnant women who are consuming alcohol, and the implementation of evidence-based interventions to reduce the risk of prenatal alcohol exposure. In addition to providing health information and advice, healthcare professionals have a responsibility to monitor and record alcohol use among all pregnant women. 'Accurate consumption histories must be taken sequentially, not retrospectively. Use of screening questionnaires (see page 16) will increase the identification of at-risk women, allowing safe drinking advice to be offered.'[82]

Monitoring and detecting maternal alcohol consumption is complicated by a number of factors including:
- an under-reporting of maternal alcohol consumption levels that can occur because women feel afraid or embarrassed to admit they are drinking during pregnancy
- embarrassment on the part of healthcare staff who view monitoring as intrusive
- the difficulty in ascertaining consumption levels in the early stages of pregnancy[h]
- inaccurately recorded patient histories of alcohol use
- poor use of screening techniques and follow-up procedures
- the lack of a reliable biological marker for maternal alcohol consumption.[9, 83-85]

There is currently no definitive test that can identify alcohol use during pregnancy or newborns exposed to alcohol prenatally. Several potentially useful biomarkers (eg fatty acid ethyl esters) are being developed that can detect varying degrees of alcohol exposure or use.[84, 86, 87] There are a number of ethical considerations for the use of these methods including the need for informed consent, the fact that

---

[9] For further information on the autonomy of pregnant women and the right to chose or reject advice or treatment please refer to *Medical Ethics Today: The BMA's Handbook of Ethics and Law (1) (1993)pp123-124.*

[h] Some women may have been drinking harmful amounts of alcohol prior to detecting their pregnancy and then will have reduced their alcohol consumption levels once they found out they were pregnant. Therefore, asking questions about their alcohol consumption levels during pregnancy may not provide accurate information regarding consumption levels during the initial stages of pregnancy.

detecting a biomarker for alcohol consumption implies a lack of trust in the information provided by the mother, and the fact that the detection process comes too late to educate and prevent harm. Further research is required to establish the validity, efficacy and ethical considerations for the use of biomarkers. Two similar routine screening methods have been specifically developed in the USA that are brief and can be used to establish alcohol use in pregnant women; the T-ACE and TWEAK alcohol screening questionnaires (see appendix 5).[88, 89] Both screening questionnaires have similar sensitivities (approximately 75%) and have been found to be efficient screening tools for identifying alcohol consumption risks during pregnancy.[4, 90-93] The T-ACE questionnaire is more specific (at 89% specificity) than the TWEAK questionnaire (at 63-83%).[91] There is some evidence that the latter may be better at identifying women who are not problem drinkers but who consume alcohol at low-to-moderate levels.[4] The T-ACE and TWEAK questionnaires are recommended by both the DH and the Scottish Intercollegiate Guidelines Network (SIGN) as simple screening tools for detecting alcohol misuse among pregnant women.[94, 95] It is important that the T-ACE and TWEAK screening questionnaires are used as part of routine antenatal screening. A number of other screening questionnaires that assess the quantity and frequency of alcohol consumption have been developed; for example the Fast Alcohol Screening Test (FAST) which is a short questionnaire that screens for hazardous drinking as well as harmful drinking and dependence.[96] These screening questionnaires are not specifically designed for use with pregnant women. Further research is required into the most effective screening method for maternal alcohol consumption in the UK.

Screening for alcohol use and misuse is not a routine component of primary care in the UK.[i] The new General Medical Services (nGMS) contract includes an optional alcohol National Enhanced Service (NES) section that aims to create a small number of more specialist GPs, who undertake basic screening and more specialist interventions. In the UK, pregnant women are routinely screened for a number of specific conditions including haematological conditions (eg anaemia), fetal anomalies (eg Down's syndrome), infections (eg rubella) and clinical conditions (eg gestational diabetes mellitus). There is, however, no routine screening system for specifically monitoring alcohol consumption during pregnancy. Screening for alcohol use and misuse should be considered as part of the routine antenatal screening tests provided to pregnant women as a part of National Health Service (NHS) care. This requires appropriate training, resources and incentives for staff. Guidance on screening for alcohol use during pregnancy is not included in the NICE guidance on antenatal care, *Routine care for the healthy pregnant women* (NICE, 2003).[97] Further guidance for healthcare professionals is required on the monitoring of and screening for alcohol use and misuse during pregnancy.

In addition to identifying at-risk pregnancies, routine antenatal screening for maternal alcohol consumption would assist in the identification of newborn children who are at greatest risk of FASD, and women most at risk of a subsequent birth of an affected child. The screening process itself would also serve to raise awareness of the dangers of maternal alcohol consumption, and it has been suggested that this alone may be related to a reduction in drinking during pregnancy.[75]

---

[i] Under the new General Medical Services (nGMS) contract, GPs are not required to provide alcohol services as part of the essential services component or through the Quality in Outcomes Framework (QOF). The QOF is a component of the nGMS that rewards practices for the provision of quality care, and helps to fund further improvements in the delivery of clinical care. Participation by practices in the QOF is voluntary. For participating practices, the QOF measures practice achievement against a range of evidence-based clinical indicators and against a range of indicators covering practice organisation and management. Practices score points according to their levels of achievement against these indicators, and practice payments are calculated from points achieved.

Recommendations
- Screening for maternal alcohol consumption via objective screening techniques such as T-ACE and TWEAK should be considered as part of routine antenatal care in the NHS. The UK health departments together with relevant NHS bodies should ensure appropriate training, resources, guidance and incentives for this routine screening are provided.
- All healthcare professionals involved in the provision of antenatal care should ensure that alcohol use among pregnant women is monitored and recorded appropriately.
- Further research should be undertaken to examine the:
  - use and validity of biological markers for detecting maternal alcohol consumption
  - ethical considerations for the use of biological markers of maternal alcohol consumption
  - most effective screening method for maternal alcohol consumption.

Referral for brief interventions

Brief interventions are intended to provide prophylactic treatment before or soon after the onset and identification of alcohol-related problems. Research has found that brief interventions produce clinically significant effects on drinking behaviour and related problems.[4, 79, 92-95] In prenatal settings, they have been shown to be a low-cost and effective method of reducing or stopping alcohol consumption during pregnancy in women who are nondependent and who consume alcohol at low-to-moderate levels.[4, 83, 90, 95] It has been found that brief interventions in pregnant women may produce improved birth and neurobehavioral outcomes in their children, and decrease alcohol consumption during subsequent pregnancies in high-risk women.[4, 90, 98] The effects of brief interventions have been found to be significantly enhanced by partner participation.[99]

Brief interventions commonly consist of a number of stages including assessment, feedback and goal setting.[4, 83] They are delivered using behavioural modification techniques and reinforced with the provision of written material. The type of brief intervention provided is dependent on the level of maternal alcohol consumption, the stage of pregnancy and the severity of dependence on alcohol. Simple brief interventions involve a specific brief interview provided by a competent practitioner immediately following a screening assessment.[94] Extended brief interventions incorporate a series of these structured interviews (between three and 12) delivered by a competent practitioner.[94] They can be delivered in a variety of settings, including medical settings – such as primary care and accident and emergency – and in generic non-specialist services. Routine antenatal care provides a useful opportunity to deliver a brief intervention for reducing alcohol consumption, as well as access to contraceptive information and services.

There is no specific guidance on the use of brief interventions in the prenatal setting. *Models of care for alcohol misusers* (DH, 2006) provides best practice guidance on the treatment of adult alcohol misusers, including information on simple and extended brief interventions. This outlines the type of advice that should be offered during a brief intervention, including:
- information about the nature and effects of alcohol and its potential for harm
- personalised feedback on risk and harm
- emphasis on the individual's personal responsibility for change
- attempts to increase the patient's confidence in being able to reduce their alcohol consumption ('self-efficacy')
- goal-setting (for example, start dates and daily or weekly targets for drinking)

- written self-help material for the individual to take away, containing more detailed information on consequences of excessive drinking and tips for cutting down (this can be in a variety of media, including electronic, such as the internet)
- signposting individuals to having a wider general health check, where indicated
- arrangements for follow-up monitoring.[94]

Further guidance is required on the referral for, and provision of, brief interventions in the antenatal setting.

Recommendations
- The UK health departments should produce specific guidance on the referral for, and provision of, brief interventions for women who are pregnant, or who are considering a pregnancy.
- Any woman who is pregnant, or who is planning a pregnancy, and who has a suspected or confirmed history of alcohol consumption at low-to-moderate levels should be offered brief intervention counselling. This should occur at the earliest possible stage and be considered a part of routine antenatal care where required.
- All healthcare professionals providing antenatal care should be trained in the delivery of brief interventions within this setting, as well as having appropriate resources to ensure this is carried out effectively.

Targeted prevention for 'at-risk' women
Where a woman is identified as being at high-risk of prenatal alcohol exposure, healthcare professionals have a responsibility to implement targeted intervention protocols. Several innovative indicated prevention strategies have been trialled in the USA (see appendix 6). These prevention efforts target women at high-risk of prenatal alcohol exposure, including those with a history of alcohol misuse, those with severe alcohol problems, and women who have previously delivered a child affected by alcohol.[75, 100] Further, the Centre for Substance Abuse Treatment (CSAT) and the Substance Abuse and Mental Health Services Administration (SAMHSA), within the US Department of Health and Human Services has produced treatment improvement protocols (TIPs). These are best practice guidelines for the treatment of substance abuse and intended to stimulate a wide variety of service providers to participate in crafting a full continuum of family-oriented services for pregnant, substance-using women and their children.[101]

There is no evidence that brief interventions are effective among individuals with more severe alcohol problems and levels of dependence.[92] Referral to specialist alcohol services should therefore be considered for women who are dependent on alcohol and who are pregnant, or those trying to conceive. Specialised treatment services consist of both therapeutic approaches (eg relapse prevention) and management components (eg detoxification facilities, inpatient residential programmes and outpatient clinics). There is no specific guidance on the referral of women at high-risk of prenatal alcohol exposure. Guidance on the referral and follow-up of patients with alcohol problems is outlined in *The management of harmful drinking and alcohol dependence in primary care* (SIGN, 2003), however, this does not provide specific guidance on problem drinking during pregnancy.[95] Further guidance is required on the referral of women at high-risk of prenatal alcohol exposure to specialist alcohol services.

Recommendations
- The UK health departments should produce specific guidance for the implementation of targeted interventions and referral to specialist alcohol services for women at high-risk of prenatal alcohol exposure, including those with a history of alcohol misuse, those with severe alcohol problems, and women who have previously had a child affected by alcohol.
- Any woman who is identified as being at high-risk of prenatal alcohol exposure should be offered referral to specialist alcohol services for appropriate treatment. Any referral should be followed up and assessed at regular intervals.

Matthew's story...

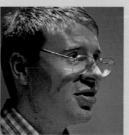 I am one of the oldest known FASD diagnosed in the UK. FASD are a part of me and I have never known any different although I think I can see what 'normal' is, although there is no definitive answer to that.

If there's a hard way to do things I usually take that route (schoolwork & employment). Get tired quite easily and quickly when bored. Also tire quickly if I have to concentrate hard on things that are unfamiliar to me. Find starting new tasks hard and have to be told more than once how to do things. Also forget and have to be retold everything.

I get very nervous and scared inside. You don't want anyone's help with anything because you feel like a loser if you ask for it and won't understand what they're on about anyhow if they do try to help you. Continually judge myself when there's no need to creating a spiral effect that increases my anxiety. I can only think of one thing at a time in one direction.

Feel, look and act much younger than I am. I fantasise about my life and often want to be the greatest person in the world. Take hours on one thing like an essay (get blocked don't know where or how to begin so just start waffling on hoping something might give me credit).

I cannot read body language so am wary of other people but very friendly towards them at the same time. I imagine how people might be feeling towards me but get the wrong impression. Good long-term and poor short-term memory – can remember things like phone numbers and car registration plates from 20 years ago but can't remember who I met this morning or did I lock the car when I left it 30 seconds ago? I cannot necessarily remember people well though.

On the outside you look normal but very few people have actually clicked with me as friends. Music helps to stimulate my brain and singing a lot makes me happy and produces adrenaline.

I used to feel angry with my natural parents and still find relations with my father difficult but don't see my mother.

I suffer from depression and from loneliness and due to this my vulnerability is increased leading to risky and frightening situations. Although I have had thoughts of suicide I am too strong to ever go through with it.

Interactions with other people are hard although rarely feel bored when on my own due to obsessive behaviour.

Government policy in the UK towards alcohol is shameful. One billion pounds per year spent in the NHS alone due to binge drinking which could be used on other affairs if FAS awareness was increased.

Management of fetal alcohol spectrum disorders

The management of the range of FASD requires a multidisciplinary approach involving a wide range of healthcare professionals – including paediatricians, obstetricians, psychologists, GPs, neurologists, psychiatrists, clinical geneticists, health visitors and midwives – as well as individuals in the fields of education and social services.[2]

Diagnosis and referral

FAS, PFAS, ARND and ARBD are difficult to diagnose. In the absence of a specific diagnostic test, diagnosis involves the application of a set of clinical criteria and the determination of a history of prenatal alcohol exposure.[4, 53] Diagnostic criteria for FAS are well established, however, and based on the presence of the characteristic set of facial features combined with growth and neurocognitive deficits. FAS can be diagnosed with or without confirmed maternal alcohol exposure. The diagnostic criteria for prenatal alcohol-related conditions other than FAS are less precise and subject to considerable debate due to a lack of available scientific evidence.[102]

The range of disorders are commonly under-diagnosed reflecting a number of factors including:
- the lack of a specific diagnostic test
- an under-reporting of maternal alcohol consumption
- the difficulty in detecting the defining features associated with FASD in neonates
- confounding factors (eg poor nutritional maternal status or polydrug use)
- the lack of knowledge and understanding of FASD among healthcare professionals that means they often do not feel competent to make a diagnosis.[5, 103]

As a consequence, diagnosis at birth is rare and usually occurs later in early childhood.[5] The difficulty of diagnosis is further complicated by the fact that many genetic and malformation syndromes (eg Williams syndrome, Cornelia de Lange syndrome, Velocardiofacial syndrome) have similar clinical characteristics to to those found in the range of FASD.[51, 104] The incidence of children affected by genetic and dysmorphic syndromes, other than FASD, is the same whether or not their mothers abused alcohol when carrying them.[51] Caution should therefore be used when diagnosing a child who presents the clinical characteristics to those found in the range of FASD, as the presenting phenotype may be caused by genetic and dysmorphic syndromes other than FASD. To do otherwise could cause unnecessary stress, social stigmatisation and feelings of guilt in the parents. To confound clinical diagnosis further, children affected by prenatal alcohol exposure may also have another genetic syndrome as a comorbidity. Diagnosis in adults is particularly challenging as physical features may change over time, there may be catch-up growth, and cumulative environmental influences may distort the evaluation of brain function. Obtaining reliable information on the adult's history and abilities may also be difficult, and may be complicated by factors including alcohol and drug abuse, and mental health problems. Diagnosis of the range of FASD therefore requires skilled clinical differentiation and a good understanding of the nature of FASD and the diagnostic techniques involved in identifying the range of conditions. It is important that there is adequate funding for the development, training and maintenance of multidisciplinary diagnostic teams in the UK.

Formal diagnosis at the earliest possible stage is paramount as it permits the implementation of early intervention and treatment programmes. Early diagnosis can also decrease the risk of additional problems commonly found in individuals affected by these disorders that result from the neurocognitive deficits (eg psychiatric problems, disrupted school experience, alcohol and drug problems).[2, 5]

'The potential for learners with FASD is variable but [their] potential can be fulfilled if the environment for teaching and learning is correct. We have seen significant improvement in pupils with FASD and enjoy their success and increased skills, fitting them for life in the wider community. The earlier the diagnosis, the earlier support networks can be put in place and learning maximised.'
Celia Dawson
Headteacher: Cricket Green School (for special needs pupils)

There is no guidance in the UK on FASD diagnosis and referral. Within the UK, specific skills in diagnosing and managing neurodevelopmental conditions could lie within regional and national tier 4 (quaternary level) (see figure 1). These services already exist and could be enhanced to provide FASD services, for example Child Learning Disability services with links to local or regional genetics clinics. Developing the skills and understanding that already exists at this level would lead to a potentially cost effective method of providing viable healthcare interventions to a regional population. The CDC has developed a framework for the identification, referral, diagnosis and treatment of FAS (see figure 2).[105] This framework refers specifically to FAS, however, and further guidance is required on the diagnosis and referral of PFAS, ARND and ARBD. There are three main components of the framework including:

1. **Initial identification** – the characteristic facial features, growth deficiencies and CNS manifestations associated with FAS commonly become evident during infancy. Infants affected by FAS may exhibit hyperactivity, poor fine-motor control, social naivety, and/or intellectual disabilities, and they may be irritable and fail to meet developmental milestones.[5] Initial recognition can be made by the child's parents, school teachers, social service professionals and healthcare professionals.

2. **Referral** – where FAS is suspected by a healthcare professional an initial evaluation is required to gather specific data on the characteristic features of FAS (facial malformations, growth abnormalities, neurodevelopmental concerns) and to determine any history of maternal alcohol use. A child who meets the specific FAS referral criteria should be referred to a specialist for a complete diagnostic evaluation.

3. **Diagnosis** – confirmed diagnosis is made by a multidisciplinary team following a thorough assessment of the child, including evaluation of dysmorphia and growth parameters, and appropriate neurodevelopmental data. The diagnostic approach includes physical examination, intelligence tests, occupational and physical therapy, and psychological, speech and neurological evaluations.

Figure 1 – proposed model for FASD service delivery based on UK current practice

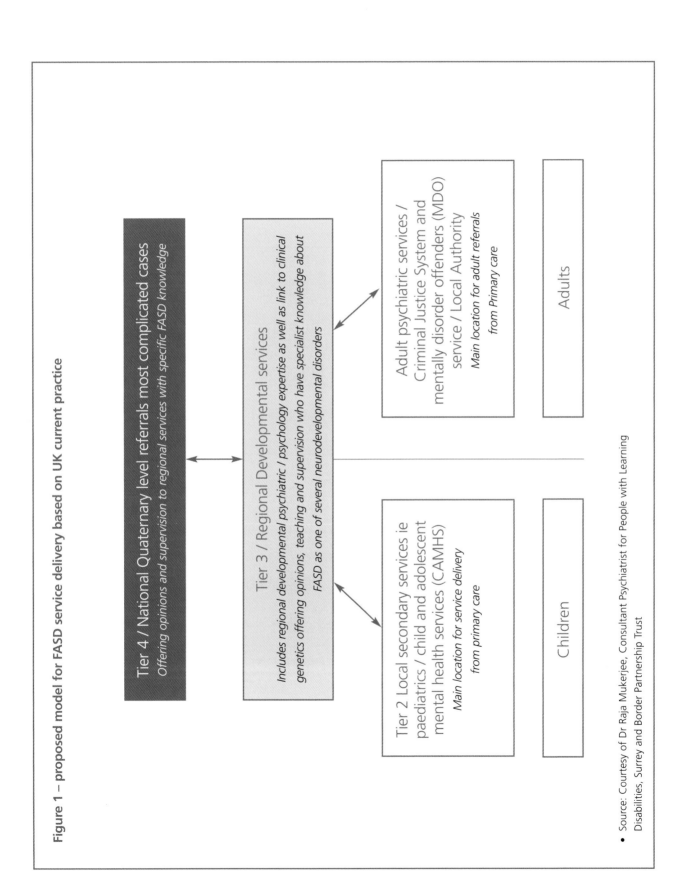

Tier 4 / National Quaternary level referrals most complicated cases
Offering opinions and supervision to regional services with specific FASD knowledge

Tier 3 / Regional Developmental services
Includes regional developmental psychiatric / psychology expertise as well as link to clinical genetics offering opinions, teaching and supervision who have specialist knowledge about FASD as one of several neurodevelopmental disorders

Adult psychiatric services / Criminal Justice System and mentally disorder offenders (MDO) service / Local Authority
Main location for adult referrals from Primary care

Adults

Tier 2 Local secondary services ie paediatrics / child and adolescent mental health services (CAMHS)
Main location for service delivery from primary care

Children

Source: Courtesy of Dr Raja Mukerjee, Consultant Psychiatrist for People with Learning Disabilities, Surrey and Border Partnership Trust

Figure 2 – the CDC framework for FAS diagnosis and follow-up care

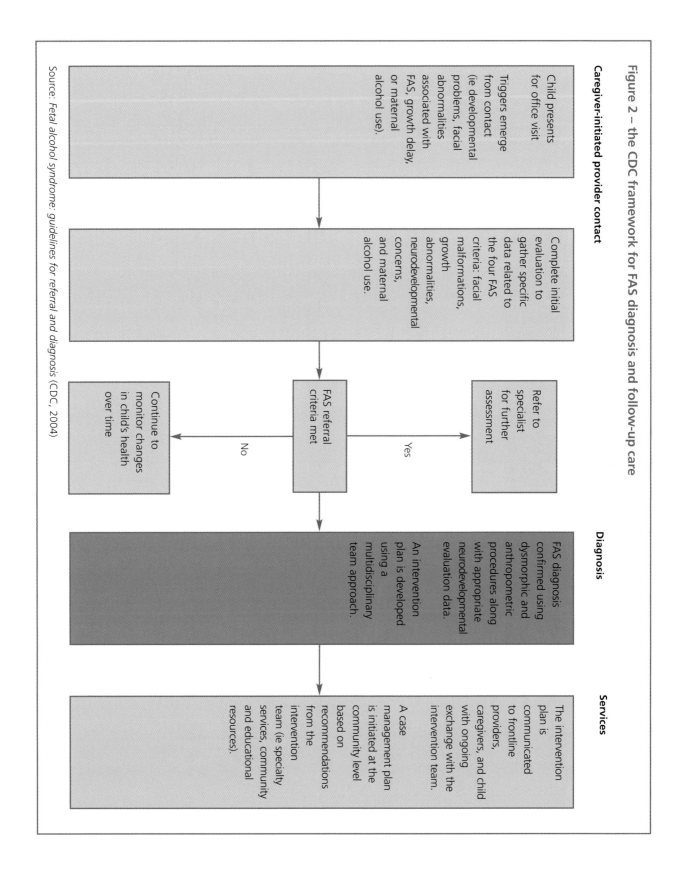

Caregiver-initiated provider contact

Child presents for office visit

Triggers emerge from contact (ie developmental problems, facial abnormalities associated with FAS, growth delay, or maternal alcohol use).

Complete initial evaluation to gather specific data related to the four FAS criteria: facial malformations, growth abnormalities, neurodevelopmental concerns, and maternal alcohol use.

FAS referral criteria met

No → Continue to monitor changes in child's health over time

Yes → Refer to specialist for further assessment

Diagnosis

FAS diagnosis confirmed using dysmorphic and anthropometric procedures along with appropriate neurodevelopmental evaluation data.

An intervention plan is developed using a multidisciplinary team approach.

Services

The intervention plan is communicated to frontline providers, caregivers, and child with ongoing exchange with the intervention team.

A case management plan is initiated at the community level based on recommendations from the intervention team (ie specialty services, community and educational resources).

There are several sets of diagnostic criteria currently used for the evaluation and categorisation of the effects of prenatal alcohol exposure. These include the Institute of Medicine (IoM) criteria (see appendix 7a) the CDC criteria (see appendix 8), the 4-Digit Diagnostic Code (see appendix 9) and the Canadian FASD guidelines (see appendix 10). A revised version of the IoM diagnostic criteria[j] has been developed in an attempt to improve the practical application of the IoM criteria in a clinical setting (see appendix 7b).[106] The diagnostic criteria vary between these different sets of guidelines. The 4-Digit Code, the Canadian FASD guidelines and the revised IoM guidelines cover the full spectrum of FASD diagnostic outcomes, while the CDC guidelines address FAS only.[107] The guidelines also differ in their criteria for FAS diagnosis. The CDC guidelines have more relaxed facial and CNS criteria compared to the 4-Digit Code and the Canadian guidelines. The revised IoM guidelines further relax the facial criteria, restrict the CNS criteria to structural abnormalities only, and require confirmed alcohol exposure to be excessive.[107]

A complete maternal history is also an important component in FASD diagnosis as it provides information on maternal factors that are associated with an increased risk of FASD (eg a history of alcohol and/or other substance abuse, a previous child with FASD).[5] Information on these maternal factors can be extremely valuable, if not essential, in FASD diagnosis, especially when there is no confirmed history of maternal alcohol use or when infants show only a few signs or symptoms of prenatal alcohol exposure. Training is required in how to obtain this information in a non-threatening and non-judgemental manner.

> **Recommendations**
> - The UK health departments should produce guidance for healthcare professionals in the UK on the identification, referral and diagnosis for the full range of FASD.
> - The UK health departments should ensure appropriate diagnostic and referral services for FASD are adequately provided and resourced throughout the UK. There should be adequate funding for the development, training and maintenance of multidisciplinary diagnostic teams.

Clinical management

There has been very little research into the clinical management of FASD,[2] and there is no framework for clinical management of FASD in the UK. After the birth of a child who has FASD there are essentially two targets for intervention: the mother and the child. Each is in need of care to treat and improve their health as well as to prevent the birth of another FASD child. Often FASD children are placed in foster care because of neglect or abuse. As such, a key reason for improving the social and health position of the mother is so that she can continue or regain care of her child(ren) as well as taking care of her health.

It is important that diagnosed individuals and their families are linked to appropriate resources and services. Effective clinical management requires the implementation of postnatal interventions and the cooperation between a wide range of healthcare professionals including GPs, obstetricians, paediatricians, psychiatrists, psychologists, and speech and language therapists (see figure 3). Further management requires specialist support in the provision of education and social services. The adverse effects of prenatal alcohol exposure on learning and life skills varies significantly among individuals, thus management programmes have to be tailored to the individual and his or her family.

---

[j] The revised IoM guidelines are commonly known as the Hoyme diagnostic guidelines.

Social services may be required to ensure a supportive and stable home environment and to provide parental education. Educational support is essential during schooling years and requires adequately trained school staff. For intervention programmes to be effective, they need to be focused on an individual's developmental level. Intervention strategies for school-age children need to focus on providing specialised educational opportunities; whereas interventions for adolescents should also focus on providing vocational and transitional services (eg employment skills). It is important that healthcare professionals work closely with education and social service providers to ensure that individuals affected by the range of FASD are appropriately assessed in terms of their communication and social skills, emotional maturity, verbal and comprehension abilities, language usage, and healthcare requirements. These assessments should be used to inform the clinical management programme. It is also important that healthcare professionals provide information on the available support services to carers and their families.

Recommendations
- The UK Health departments should develop a framework for the clinical management of individuals affected by the range of FASD, as well as their birth mothers. This should be adequately resourced.
- Further research should be undertaken to examine the clinical management of individuals affected by FASD and the support systems available in the UK to them and their carers and families.

Figure 2 – timeline of aspects of management from preconception to adulthood

Time period	Pre-conception	During pregnancy	Childhood 0-18	Adult 18+
Actions to take	1 Public education 2 Pre-conception advice	1 Monitoring of pregnancy 2 Ongoing advice 3 Information documentation 4 Correspondence with colleagues	1 Early recognition 2 Diagnosis 3 Psychometric assessment 4 Educational statement (if required) 5 Ongoing support as needed 6 Physical investigations 7 Behavioural management eg ADHD symptoms 8 Further prevention	1 Diagnosis 2 Psychometric assessment 3 Physical investigation if not previously undertaken 4 Investigation of background and history from/about birth mother if possible 5 Education of others as to level of function 6 Ongoing support 7 Social 8 Financial 9 Educational 10 Employment 11 Management of secondary disabilities
Responsible practitioners	1 Government/FAS specialists 2 GP 3 Addiction psychiatrist	1 GP 2 Midwife 3 Obstetrician 4 Addiction psychiatrist	1 GP 2 Health visitor 3 Hospital paediatrician 4 Community paediatrician 5 Child psychiatrist/team 6 FAS specialist 7 Clinical geneticist 8 Addiction psychiatrist 9 Neurology 10 Public health 11 Education services	GP Clinical genetics FAS specialist Neurology Public health Community mental health teams General psychiatry Learning disability psychiatry Addiction psychiatry Forensic psychiatry Psychology Speech and language therapist Social Services Government

Psychometric, physical investigations and other recommended tests

1 IQ eg WISC/WAIS/NART

2 Executive function, eg Delis Kaplan test

3 Communication assessment

4 Brain imaging for microcephaly below 3rd percentile, midline abnormalities and from areas of decreased attenuation

5 Physical examination for cardiac, renal and orobuccal pathology

Source: Mukherjee RAS, Hollnis S & Turk J (2006) Fetal alcohol spectrum disorder: an overview. *Journal of the Royal Society of Medicine* **99**: 298-302.

Janet's story...

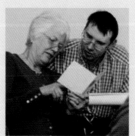 In 1978 our family fostered Matthew. He was four months old when he arrived at our home. His family had been under supervision due to his mother's bouts of alcoholism. After his birth the mother's drinking continued and Matthew and two older children were taken into care, Matthew was two weeks old. Matthew was a very sickly, quiet baby, he never cried. He was a very difficult feeder, very withdrawn, no smiles, no expressions; looking back at my notes I see that he first laughed when he was over a year old.

Matthew was diagnosed with FAS in July 1978, also a heart murmur, suspect clicky hips and flat feet. We were told that Matthew was backward and would never live a normal life. He was unable to sit up unsupported until over two years old, walked at around four years old and was only out of nappies a matter of weeks before he started school. He hardly spoke and an intensive programme to improve his language was initiated at around three years old. Matthew was a very small, vulnerable timid child. He had a small head, no body fat, indistinct features, bad coordination, poor eyesight, fragmented vision in one eye, teeth in unusual places and he hated loud noises. He also had difficulty in sleeping, was hyperactive and prone to infections – we loved him.

Matthew's play was obsessive, lines of stones, circles with string, swinging on the swing for hours whilst blowing a whistle and an extremely deep interest in windscreen wipers.

When Matthew was five he attended the local primary school, he was a very lonely and frightened little boy, no friends and isolated in the playground. He suffered agonies away from home and constantly sucked his thumb. If there was statementing at his school we were never offered it.

Matthew's first teacher at school, seeing his distress and isolation at playtimes, took him into the classroom and taught him to read which was a great achievement for Matthew. Once Matthew had learnt to read and write his obsessive play changed, he made lists, hundreds of them.

The opportunity came to adopt Matthew when he was seven. Matthew continued on with his education, in some areas he appeared bright, in others no ability at all and no aptitude for any sport. Fantasy was second nature to Matthew and this is something that continues to this day.

At eleven he started at the secondary school which was a nightmare for him. I used to have to walk him to school as he was unsure of the way and leave him at the corner by the school. He was very lost and confused and lonely. He was unable to find his way around the school and not finding the toilets for several days.

Matthew is very stoical and endured his days there. He experienced a breakdown or a form of panic attack when he was 12 and a Social Services Counsellor was called in by the school.

My husband's job sent us to Hong Kong when Matthew had turned 12 and we were there for almost four years. This was a mainly successful time for Matthew. I have read that there is a learning opportunity for children with FASD around the age of 13 and so this proved with Matthew. He attended an international school and learnt much which he still enjoys today.

cont...

From the ages of 13 to 16 he learnt to canoe, bike ride round the territory, sing in a choir, become involved in stage management, improve his swimming and gain three GCSEs. He really loved his time there and achieved much although during our stay he saw a psychiatrist and had counselling for inappropriate behaviour. One of the findings from these sessions was his inability to recognise body language and facial expressions.

Throughout his teens we always had to remind Matthew to shave, wash, change clothes etc. He had a checklist on his bedroom door to consult before he left in the morning. Sleep patterns were still poor and he slept with the radio on and still does. He achieved much but almost always took the more difficult route.

He worked very hard and achieved a BTEC in Performing Arts. Obviously it was difficult for Matthew to work in stage management; jobs were few and far between and he was also very immature for his age.

He got himself a six month web design course where he was paid a small salary. He was saving for driving lessons as he needed a British driving licence; his main ambition was to drive. He was still lonely, craving excessive physical contact, hugs and kisses something which had been ongoing his whole life; also when troubled he developed a childlike voice, and sucked his thumb.

At the age of 22 years old it was felt the time had come for Matthew to begin to live on his own with support from his parents. He began a new job and together we found him a room in a house, from there he biked to his job. It was a very difficult time for Matthew, difficulty with time keeping and trying to understand his job and live away from the family.

Matthew was always good with money, he wouldn't starve although when the supermarket layout was altered he came home without any food and eventually I discovered this and had to go with him and show him the new layout; it's all these little complications that make life difficult for him.

It soon became clear that Matthew couldn't cope with his job, the inability to begin new tasks and poor social skills all contributed to this. We had also at this time sought help from the Social Services. It was difficult to get any help as Matthew didn't seem to fall within any category. No one seemed to have any idea of the needs of a young adult with FASD.

Finally appointments were made for Matthew to see a consultant psychiatrist for learning difficulties. Also an occupational therapist, who carried out some very valuable sessions with Matthew teaching him how to read body language and facial expressions from photographs.

Work continued to be a problem, he was given less to do as he made mistakes, his self esteem was low and he was feeling ill from the Seroxat. Matthew is very determined, he wanted to feel well so with advice from his GP he gradually reduced his dosage over a period of months until he was off them completely.

Work was not improving and we were at a loss as to how to advise him, we feared that if Matthew became unemployed he would be at risk. The disability job adviser tried to help but nothing improved. I can't tell you how many agencies I have sought help and advice from over the years without any results, most not having any idea what I am talking about.

cont...

He was unhappy and lonely, spent a large amount of time sleeping. He had previously gone into chat rooms on the internet and we had warned him of the dangers of this. Suddenly Matthew seemed busy and more content, we should have been warned. Then we received a phone call from Matthew saying he was being blackmailed for £5,000. He had become involved via a chat room with a young man who, unbeknown to him, was a drug addict. After a few weeks of supposed friendship he demanded money with threats to harm Matthew. This culminated in the young man forcing his way into Matthew's flat. Matthew had been beaten up, held at knife point, handcuffed and sexually assaulted throughout the night. Matthew had stayed calm, managed to escape, called the police and seen the young man arrested. Matthew had several vulnerable persons interviews with the police, his father accompanied him.

All this agony for Matthew is because he is lonely, can't read body language, has low self esteem and is immature for his age, this is due to FASD.

Due to this assault Matthew had to move flats and now he has a quiet flat in a complex with an alarm call. The Social Services found this for him. Matthew passed his driving test after six attempts and he bought a car. This has made a big difference to Matthew, he is now independent, he drives everywhere. His job had become non-existent; he was bullied and sworn at.

We went to see a new young GP who knew about FASD, the first time we haven't had to explain anything. The next question was whether his job was supported. He treated Matthew for depression and gave him sick leave and then, later put him on incapacity benefit; he shows great interest in Matthew and wants to help him.

After a month's wait we saw the disability job adviser, and [Matthew] was offered a course aimed at getting him back into work. He could attend at his own pace, he would be assessed and suitable employment would be found for him and he would be supported within the workplace. He is now 29 years old and he is hopeful.

As Matthew said once he had left his job, 'Maybe it's all for the best Mum' what amazing young people they are with FASD.

I always speak the truth to Matthew, I tell it as it is. It can be painful and difficult for both of us but it must be so. I have always tried to stand back and let Matthew go, he sometimes makes mistakes, so do I. He's only just beginning to grow into his age.

The one thing that worries my husband and myself is the lack of a circle of support for Matthew outside the family, very necessary as we get older and eventually die.

I have nothing but admiration for Matthew, he has had many hurdles to climb, dreadful things have happened to him but he just picks himself up and tries again. He is a survivor; at last his head is up, he now stands straight. His father and I are very proud to be his parents.

Conclusions

The range of FASD are a significant health consequence of maternal alcohol consumption that can cause immense distress and personal difficulties to those affected. The effects of prenatal alcohol exposure are complex and can range from mild cognitive impairment to the full presentation of FAS that is characterised by facial dysmorphology, growth deficiencies and neurocognitive deficits. The range of disorders is not adequately recognised in the UK and internationally. While FAS is now widely accepted as a clearly diagnosable disorder, the clinical features of PFAS, ARND and ARBD are less well defined and subject to considerable debate. As a consequence, the epidemiology of the full range of disorders is not accurately known. Emerging data suggest that the incidences of FASD are higher than previously estimated and that some populations, including those which experience high degrees of social deprivation and poverty, are more likely to have children affected by the range of FASD.[16-20] In the UK, data on the incidences of FASD are extremely limited and, are restricted to FAS. It is vital that efforts are made to establish the epidemiology of the range of FASD in the UK through an increased recognition of these disorders, improved data collection and UK-based research.

Accurate information regarding the risks of alcohol consumption during pregnancy is necessary for the implementation of health promotion and prevention strategies. While the exact mechanisms of alcohol teratogenesis remain uncertain, it is clear that heavy maternal alcohol consumption can adversely impact on fetal development and lead to significant postnatal and long-term problems for the child. The occurrence of FAS has been found to be strongly associated with heavy maternal alcohol use – particularly in cases of alcohol dependence or severe alcohol problems – and with the frequency of heavy dose drinking.[4, 5, 14, 43] These findings are significant given the substantial rise in recent years in the number of women of childbearing age in the UK who engage in heavy and/or binge drinking, and the frequency of unplanned pregnancies. The causal relationships between maternal alcohol consumption and PFAS, ARBD and ARND are less well understood. It is clear that individuals affected by PFAS, ARBD and/or ARND exhibit some, but not all, of the anomalies found in individuals affected by FAS. Research has shown there to be critical periods of fetal development that are particularly sensitive to the effects of prenatal alcohol exposure at heavy doses.[2, 4, 5, 41] It has been suggested that the anomalies associated with PFAS, ARBD and ARND may result from exposure to heavy doses of alcohol during specific periods of fetal development whereas FAS results from exposure to heavy doses throughout a pregnancy.[43]

There is considerable debate as to the adverse effects of prenatal alcohol exposure at low-to-moderate levels as the existing evidence is inconclusive. Research evidence is continuing to emerge as to the potential effects of prenatal alcohol exposure at low-to-moderate levels,[52-61] however, it is currently not possible to predict who is and is not at risk. Given the ambiguity regarding the level of individual risk to the developing fetus and the fact that health promotion advice and sensible drinking guidelines lack clarity, the only sure way to prevent these disorders is to stop alcohol consumption during pregnancy.

Preventing the adverse impact of alcohol consumption during pregnancy remains a significant challenge, not least because of the poor levels of awareness and understanding of FASD among healthcare professionals and the general public. Effective universal prevention strategies necessitate the implementation of policies that alter drinking behaviour. Controlling the price and availability of alcohol are effective determinants of drinking behaviour that need to be considered as part of any public health strategy aimed at reducing drinking during pregnancy. The use of health promotion and educational programmes have been shown to be ineffective at altering drinking behaviour and must therefore be considered as part of a wider alcohol-harm reduction strategy. The primary and community care settings provide the ideal opportunity to deliver selective prevention strategies including screening for maternal alcohol consumption and referral for brief intervention. Targeted prevention strategies for women who are at high-risk of having children affected by FASD include treatment of alcohol addiction problems (ie referral to specialist alcohol services) and family planning advice so as to prevent the risk of having a FASD affected child.[100]

The management of FASD incorporates the identification, referral, diagnosis and treatment of individuals affected by prenatal exposure to alcohol. Early diagnosis is vital to ensure appropriate treatment and support systems are implemented at the earliest stage. The lack of knowledge and understanding of FASD among healthcare professionals means they often do not feel competent to make a diagnosis. This is compounded by the absence of validated diagnostic or screening tools, the under-reporting of maternal alcohol consumption, the difficulty in detecting the defining features of FASD, and the similarity between the characteristic features of FASD and other genetic and malformation syndromes. As a consequence, FASD are rarely diagnosed at birth or in infancy. There is a lack of specific guidance on diagnosis, referral and treatment in the UK. Several sets of diagnostic criteria have been developed to assist in the evaluation and categorisation of the effects of prenatal alcohol exposure. It is important that similar systems are adopted in the UK to ensure individuals affected by FASD are effectively identified. A greater emphasis is required on the clinical management of individuals affected by FASD through further research and the development of appropriate guidance. Treatment for FASD requires the implementation of tailored management programmes and specialised support in the provision of healthcare, education and social services.

For a range of conditions that are entirely preventable, an increased awareness among the general public and healthcare professionals together with improved clinical guidelines for the prevention and management of FASD are effective means of tackling this growing concern.

Recommendations

Combating the health consequences associated with FASD will require a multi-agency, multi-factoral approach. More research is essential so that there can be clarity to patients and healthcare professionals alike, and so that interventions can be based upon an evidence base. The recommendations to follow demonstrate the paucity of research, evidence and 'joined-up' action at present.

Healthcare professionals

- All healthcare professionals as a part of routine clinical care should provide ongoing advice and support to expectant mothers at every stage of pregnancy and this should include the risks of maternal alcohol consumption.

- All health promotion and advice should be supplemented with 'take home' printed information on the risks of consuming alcohol during pregnancy. Printed information should be:
  - clear and concise
  - available for all healthcare professionals and primary care organisations to use
  - reviewed to ensure that they are targeted at the population at risk, including difficult to reach groups.

- All healthcare professionals involved in the provision of antenatal care should ensure that alcohol use among pregnant women is monitored and recorded appropriately.

- Any woman who is pregnant, or who is planning a pregnancy, and who has a suspected or confirmed history of alcohol consumption at low-to-moderate levels should be offered brief intervention counselling. This should occur at the earliest possible stage and be considered a part of routine antenatal care where required.

- Any woman who is identified as being at high-risk of prenatal alcohol exposure should be offered referral to specialist alcohol services for appropriate treatment. Any referral should be followed up and assessed at regular intervals.

UK health departments

- The UK health departments should:
  - ensure data on FAS are routinely collected throughout the UK and consider how this should be extended to cover the range of FASD
  - implement training programmes for healthcare professionals on the prevention, diagnosis and management of the range of FASD
  - work in partnership with relevant stakeholder organisations to revise current guidance on sensible drinking (see appendix 3). They should ensure that consistent and clear advice is given to healthcare professionals and the general public regarding the sensible drinking message and the risks of alcohol consumption during pregnancy
  - produce specific guidance on the referral for, and provision of, brief interventions for women who are pregnant, or who are considering a pregnancy
  - produce specific guidance for the implementation of targeted interventions and referral to specialist alcohol services for women at high-risk of prenatal alcohol exposure, including those with a history of alcohol misuse, those with severe alcohol problems, and women who have previously had a child affected by alcohol
  - produce guidance for healthcare professionals in the UK on the identification, referral and diagnosis for the full range of FASD
  - ensure appropriate diagnostic and referral services for FASD are adequately provided and resourced throughout the UK. There should be adequate funding for the development, training and maintenance of multidisciplinary diagnostic teams

- develop a framework for the clinical management of individuals affected by the range of FASD, as well as their birth mothers. This should be adequately resourced.

- Screening for maternal alcohol consumption via objective screening techniques such as T-ACE and TWEAK should be considered as part of routine antenatal care in the NHS. The UK health departments together with relevant NHS bodies should ensure appropriate training, resources, guidance and incentives for this routine screening are provided.

- All healthcare professionals providing antenatal care should be trained in the delivery of brief interventions within this setting, as well as having appropriate resources to ensure this is carried out effectively.

- The UK government should review existing alcohol control policies in the UK to ensure that they are evidence-based and effective. This should include the introduction of increased taxation on alcohol products and the implementation of policies limiting the availability of alcohol. Any changes to existing alcohol control policies should be regularly reviewed and evaluated.

- Health promotion, and public and school-based educational programmes aimed at preventing FASD should only be used as part of a wider alcohol-related harm reduction strategy to support other policies that are effective at altering drinking behaviour.

Sensible drinking guidelines
- Women who are pregnant, or who are considering a pregnancy, should be advised not to consume any alcohol.

Research
- Research should be undertaken to:
  - determine the current levels of understanding and knowledge of the range of FASD among healthcare professionals in the UK
  - establish current public attitudes and levels of awareness of FASD in the UK and the risks of alcohol consumption during pregnancy among the general public.

- Further research should be undertaken to:
  - establish the epidemiology of the range of FASD in the UK through an increased recognition of these disorders, improved data collection and UK-based research. This should build on existing data and highlight the differences in populations through coordinated large-scale national and international studies
  - examine the relationship between prenatal alcohol exposure and the range of conditions associated with FASD. This research should build on existing work in this area and occur via population screening that is based on an active ascertainment process
  - clarify the exact mechanisms of ethanol teratogenesis and establish how they relate to the pattern of anomalies associated with FASD
  - identify the most effective ways to educate the public about the range of FASD and to alter drinking behaviour. This requires systematic studies that compare various universal prevention strategies and their impacts across the different social groups
  - examine the use and validity of biological markers for detecting maternal alcohol consumption
  - consider the ethical considerations for the use of biological markers of maternal alcohol consumption
  - establish the most effective screening method for maternal alcohol consumption
  - examine the clinical management of individuals affected by FASD and the support systems available in the UK to them and their carers and families.

Further information

This listing of organisations and publications is intended for further information only. The BMA is not responsible for the content or accuracy of external websites, nor does it endorse or otherwise guarantee the veracity of statements made in non-BMA publications.

FASD organisations
National Organisation on Fetal Alcohol Syndrome (NOFAS-UK)
www.nofas-uk.org
NOFAS-UK promotes public awareness about the risks of alcohol consumption during pregnancy with the goal to reduce the number of babies being born with FASD. It further acts as a source of information to the general public, press and to medical professionals.

National Organisation on Fetal Alcohol Syndrome (NOFAS-USA)
www.nofas.org

FAS Aware UK
www.fasaware.co.uk
This website has been designed to raise awareness, give informed choice, provide information and support for people affected by / interested in FAS.

FASD Connections
www.fasdconnections.ca/index.htm
FASD Connections is committed to building a community in which adolescents and adults with FASD are included and encouraged and where their desire and potential is supported; where the experience of families is understood, acknowledged, and accepted; and where systems are equipped to respond in an informed, compassionate and responsible way.

Fetal Alcohol Syndrome (FAS) Resources
www.esmerel.org/specific/fas.htm
This page is for disability resources that are dedicated to fetal alcohol syndrome.

Patient information resources on sensible drinking during pregnancy
- *Routine antenatal care for healthy pregnant women: understanding NICE guidance – information for pregnant women, their families and the public* (NICE, 2003)[108]
- *How much is too much? Pregnancy and Alcohol* (DH, 2006)[109]
- *Alcofacts – a guide to sensible drinking* (NHS Scotland, 2003)[110]
- NHS Health Scotland internet resource *Ready, Steady, Baby* (accessible at www.hebs.scot.nhs.uk)
- Focus on alcohol – a guide to drinking and health (HPA Northern Ireland, 2006)[111]
- The NHS funded Clinical Knowledge Summaries (CKS) service provides a patient information leaflet on pregnancy and alcohol (accessible at www.prodigy.nhs.uk)
- MIDIRS (Midwives Information and Resource Service) provides the leaflet *Informed choice: alcohol and pregnancy* (accessible at www.infochoice.org)

Providers of treatment, support and advice for people with alcohol addiction

Alcoholics anonymous

www.alcoholics-anonymous.org.uk

Alcoholics anonymous is a fellowship of men and women who share their experiences with each other so that they may solve their common problem and help others to recover from alcoholism. The only requirement for membership is a desire to stop drinking.

Alcohol concern

www.alcoholconcern.org.uk/servlets/home

Alcohol concern is the national agency on alcohol misuse. They work to reduce the incidence and costs of alcohol-related harm and to increase the range and quality of services available to people with alcohol-related problems.

Alateen

www.al-anon.org/alateen.html

Alateen is a fellowship of young Al-Anon members, usually teenagers, whose lives have been affected by someone else's drinking.

Drink and drugs.net

www.drinkanddrugs.net

The web portal for practitioners working with people with drug and alcohol problems. This site is maintained by the Federation of Drug & Alcohol Professionals (FDAP).

UK Health Departments

Department of Health

www.dh.gov.uk

The Department of Health is committed to improving the quality and convenience of care provided by the NHS and social services. Its work includes setting national standards, shaping the direction of health and social care services and promoting healthier living.

Scottish Executive Health Department (SEHD)

www.sehd.scot.nhs.uk

SEHD is responsible both for NHSScotland and for the development and implementation of health and community care policy.

The Department of Health, Social Services and Public Safety

www.dhsspsni.gov.uk

The Department's mission is to improve the health and social well-being of the people of Northern Ireland. It endeavours to do so by ensuring the provision of appropriate health and social care services, both in clinical settings, such as hospitals and GPs' surgeries, and in the community, through nursing, social work and other professional services.

NHS sites

These are the gateways to NHS services in the UK containing links to the hospital services, GP surgeries and clinics, Strategic Health Authorities / Health Boards and agencies and central government healthcare services. There is advice about healthy lifestyles, the latest local, national and international health news and online access to medical databases.

NHS England

www.nhs.uk/england/default.aspx

NHS Scotland

www.show.scot.nhs.uk

NHS Wales

www.wales.nhs.uk

Health & Social Care Services in Northern Ireland

www.healthandcareni.co.uk

NHS Direct

www.nhsdirect.nhs.uk

NHS Direct is at the forefront of 24-hour health care – delivering telephone and e-health information services day and night direct to the public.

The National Institute for Health and Clinical Excellence (NICE)

www.nice.org.uk

NICE is the independent organisation responsible for providing national guidance on the promotion of good health and the prevention and treatment of ill health.

Health Protection Agency (HPA)

www.hpa.org.uk

The HPA's role is to provide an integrated approach to protecting UK public health through the provision of support and advice to the NHS, local authorities, emergency services, other Arms Length Bodies, the Department of Health and the Devolved Administrations.

The Health Promotion Agency for Northern Ireland (HPA)

www.healthpromotionagency.org.uk

The HPA aims to provide leadership, strategic direction and support, where possible, to all those involved in promoting health in Northern Ireland.

Medical Royal Colleges

The Royal College of General Practitioners (RCGP)

www.rcgp.org.uk

The RCGP is the academic organisation in the UK for general practitioners. Its aim is to encourage and maintain the highest standards of general medical practice and act as the 'voice' of general practitioners on education, training and standards issues.

The Royal College of Paediatrics and Child Health (RCPCH)

www.rcpch.ac.uk

The RCPCH have a major role in postgraduate medical education and professional standards: setting syllabuses for postgraduate training in paediatrics, overseeing the training, running examinations, organising courses and conferences, issuing guidance and conducting research.

Royal College of Obstetricians and Gynaecologists (RCOG)

www.rcog.org.uk

The RCOG improves and maintains proper standards in the practice of obstetrics and gynaecology for the benefit of the public. The College produces evidence-based guidelines for appropriate practice and procedures, publishes patient information, books and journals and provides a range of educational tools in all aspects of obstetrics and gynaecology.

Appendix 1: characteristics associated with FASD

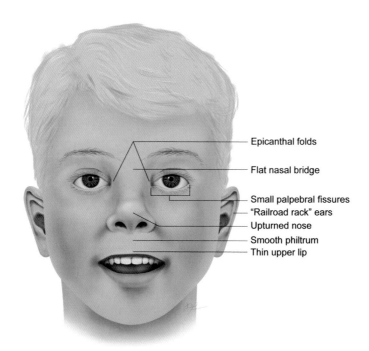

- Epicanthal folds
- Flat nasal bridge
- Small palpebral fissures
- "Railroad rack" ears
- Upturned nose
- Smooth philtrum
- Thin upper lip

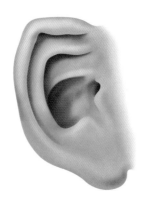

Characteristic features of an ear of a child with fetal alcohol spectrum disorders. Note the underdeveloped upper part of the ear parallel to the ear crease below ("railroad track" appearance).

Characteristic features of a hand of a child with fetal alcohol spectrum disorders. Note the curved fifth finger (clinodactyly) and the upper palmar crease that widens and ends between the second and third fingers ("hockey stick" crease).

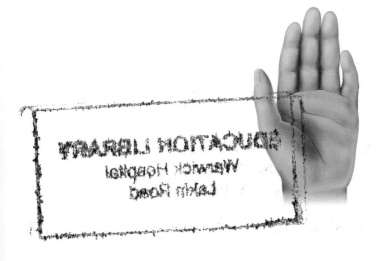

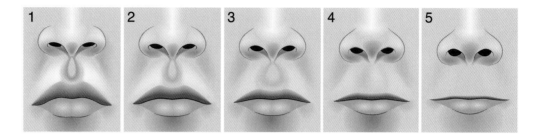

Lip-Philtrum Guide. *(A)* The smoothness of the philtrum and the thinness of the upper lip are assessed individually on a scale of 1 to 5 (1 = unaffected, 5 = most severe). The patient must have a relaxed facial expression, because a smile can alter lip thinness and philtrum smoothness. Scores of 4 and 5, in addition to short palpebral fissures, correspond to fetal alcohol syndrome.

Source: Wattendorf DJ and Muenke (2005) Fetal alcohol spectrum disorders. *American Family Physician* **72**: 279-85

Pictures courtesy of Darryl Leja, National Genome Research Institute, National Institutes of Health, Bethesda, MD.

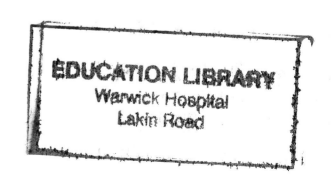

Appendix 2: maternal alcohol consumption and fetal behaviour

The effects of alcohol consumption during pregnancy have been extensively studied with respect to the individual after birth. Very few studies have focused on the adverse effects on the fetus. It is widely accepted that consumption of alcohol by women during their pregnancy may result in adverse affects on the child's health and wellbeing after birth.[41] There is little dispute that these effects result from exposure to alcohol while in the womb and that the neurobehavioural effects result from some influence of alcohol on the development and functioning of the individual's CNS. It is a matter of debate how much alcohol is required before the effects of exposure are found. Recent advances in studying the function of the fetus's CNS through observation of its behaviour may enable an assessment to be made of the levels of alcohol that adversely affect development.

Fetal behaviour can be defined as any observable action or reaction (to an external stimulus) by the fetus.[112] The behaviour may be spontaneous, that is endogenously generated by the fetus itself, or elicited, that is occurs in response to an external stimulus.[k] Observing fetal behaviour using real-time, 4-Dimensional ultrasound offers the opportunity to assess the influence of exposure to alcohol on the functioning of the fetus's brain and CNS.[112-114] Observing behaviour enables a direct assessment of any adverse effect rather than relying on statements concerning consumption.[112]

Case studies have reported that chronic and acute consumption of alcohol at high levels disrupts the normal behaviour patterns exhibited by the fetus.[115, 116] There have been few studies examining the behaviour of the fetus following acute maternal consumption of low levels of alcohol. These have been conducted in late gestation (36 weeks) and all consistently reported that consumption of alcohol exerts an immediate effect on behaviour through a rapid decrease in fetal breathing movements, lasting for two hours or more.[55-58] The more alcohol that was consumed the longer the period that breathing movements were decreased.[55-58] These studies demonstrate the potential for small amounts of alcohol, one to two glasses, to influence the behaviour of the fetus. One study examined this in more detail and observed reduced fetal eye movements, and as a consequence the behavioural state organisation of the fetus was disrupted.[58] These studies demonstrate that acute exposure to small amounts of alcohol (eg one to two units) rapidly suppresses the behaviour of the fetus and influences the functioning of the fetus's nervous system in the short term. There can be no doubt of the potential for alcohol to influence the functioning of the fetus's nervous system. The question remains as to what levels and duration of consumption are required before a permanent effect on the nervous system occurs.

---

[k] The first spontaneous movements of the fetus are observed around 7-8 weeks of gestation and are slow movements that appear to begin in the back or spine and may result in the passive displacement of the arms and legs. A wide range of movements subsequently develop and by about 20 weeks gestation the fetus exhibits most of the movements that it will produce during its time in utero, and exhibits motor patterns similar to those observed in pre-term and term infants. In terms of elicited movements, the fetus first responds to auditory stimuli at around 24-26 weeks of gestation and to visual stimuli at 26-28 weeks gestation.

The chronic (permanent) effects of alcohol on fetal behaviour have been demonstrated in a series of studies of pregnant women drinking low-to-medium levels of alcohol but who had no alcohol in their body at the time of observation (ie the effects did not result from acute alcohol exposure).[59, 60] These studies observed both spontaneous and elicited fetal startle responses.[i] An initial study found that at 27 weeks of gestation fetuses of mothers who drank alcohol exhibited a greater number of spontaneous startles but were less likely to exhibit a startle to an external stimulus than fetuses of mothers who did not drink alcohol.[59] The mean number of units of alcohol consumed by women in the study was 2.43+/- 1.37 per week, and there was no correlation between the amount drunk and effects on the fetus.[59] A second study found that exposure to alcohol increased the incidence of startle behaviour across gestation but that it appeared to delay the decrease in the incidence of startles observed with development.[60] Mothers who consumed alcohol in this study consumed an average of 4.2 +/-1.9 units of alcohol per week. As development progressed, the behaviour of those fetuses exposed to alcohol caught up with that of fetuses not exposed to alcohol.[60] At 35 weeks gestation, however, even though there was a significant catch up, the number of startles exhibited was still significantly different; with fetuses of mothers exposed to alcohol exhibiting more spontaneous startles than fetuses of mothers not exposed to alcohol.[60] These findings demonstrate that chronic consumption at low levels of exposure (ie two to five units per week) delay the development of the fetus's nervous system and may result in a permanent effect.

The observations have a number of implications for determining the best advice to be given to women during their pregnancy. Studies of acute exposure indicate that the fetus is affected by even one glass of alcohol in the short term. Thus it is not possible to say that one glass of alcohol does not affect the fetus. Moreover, there appears to be a dose dependent effect in that any effect on behaviour persists for longer at higher doses of alcohol exposure. How this relates to the neurobehavioural effects observed after birth is unknown. Other studies examining chronic effects of low dose alcohol exposure (three to five drinks/week) indicate that this does induce a delay in the fetus's behavioural development, which may catch up during gestation, but never quite reaches the levels of development exhibited by fetuses not exposed to alcohol.

---

[i] Fetal startle responses appear as rapid movements of the body lasting about one second that can occur spontaneously or in response to a stimulus. Both spontaneous and elicited startles are influenced by the development of the nervous system. Spontaneous fetal startles emerge at approximately eight weeks of pregnancy and decrease in incidence after approximately nine weeks of gestation. Elicited startle responses occur later in pregnancy (from approximately 24 to 26 weeks gestation) and become more developed (ie occur more rapidly and directly following presentation of a stimulus) as the nervous system develops.

Appendix 3: current UK guidelines on alcohol consumption during pregnancy

Guidance source	Recommendation
Department of Health (DH) *Sensible drinking* (DH, 1995)	'Women who are trying to become pregnant or are at any stage of pregnancy, should not drink more than one or two units of alcohol once or twice a week, and should avoid episodes of intoxication.'[117]
Prime Minister's Strategy Unit (PMSU) *Alcohol harm reduction strategy for England* (PMSU, 2004)	'Some groups, such as pregnant women and those engaging in potentially dangerous activities (such as operating heavy machinery), should drink less or nothing at all.'[118]
National Institute for Health and Clinical Excellence (NICE) *Antenatal care: routine care for the healthy pregnant woman* (NICE, 2003)	'Excess alcohol has an adverse effect on the fetus. Therefore it is suggested that women limit alcohol consumption to no more than one standard unit per day. Each of the following constitutes one 'unit' of alcohol: a single measure of spirits, one small glass of wine, and a half pint of ordinary strength beer, lager or cider.'[97]
Health Promotion Agency (HPA) for Northern Ireland *Focus on alcohol – a guide to drinking and health* (HPA, 2006)	'Alcohol can damage an unborn baby, so women who are pregnant should avoid alcohol, or at least cut down to a couple of drinks a week. Couples who are trying to get pregnant should also cut down, as alcohol can affect both the egg and the cells which produce sperm.'[111]
National Health Service (NHS) Health Scotland *Alcofacts – a guide to sensible drinking* (NHS Health Scotland, 2003)	'If you are pregnant or trying to become pregnant, you should not drink more than one or two units of alcohol, once or twice a week. Some doctors think it is best not to drink at all.'[110]
Scottish Executive Health Department *Hidden harm – next steps* (Scottish Executive 2006)	'Drug and alcohol use should be routinely recorded at ante-natal clinics and linked to stillbirths, congenital abnormalities and subsequent developmental abnormalities. At present, national statistics on drug use in pregnancy are available from the maternity record (SMR02) and the Scottish Birth Record (SBR). Evidence suggests that current practice in recording this information is variable. In order to improve the recording of these data and the detection of problem drug and alcohol use in pregnancy, research into current practices is being commissioned.' 'Linked to this is the development of the Scottish Women Held Maternity Record and its associated electronic record, which should also contribute to a more accurate and consistent recording of this information; and the use of appropriate screening tools to improve the detection and treatment of alcohol problems within pre- and antenatal settings.'
Royal College of Obstetricians and Gynaecologists (RCOG) *Alcohol consumption and the outcomes of pregnancy* (RCOG, 2006)	'There is an increasing body of evidence suggesting harm to the fetus from alcohol consumption during pregnancy. While the safest approach may be to avoid any alcohol intake during pregnancy, it remains the case that there is no evidence of harm from low levels of alcohol consumption, defined as no more than one or two units of alcohol once or twice a week.'[51]

Appendix 4: alcohol-related harm reduction strategies in the UK

In England, the strategy for communicating information on alcohol was set out in *Alcohol harm reduction strategy for England* (PMSU, 2004) which outlined the plans to overhaul the way that government provides information on alcohol consumption, based on the sensible drinking message.[118] This was re-enforced in *Choosing health: making healthier choices easier* (DH, 2004).[119] The harm reduction strategy incorporated a series of measures including making the sensible drinking message easier to understand and apply, targeting messages at those most at risk (including binge and chronic drinkers), providing better information for consumers both on products, and at the point of sale, and providing alcohol education in schools that can change attitudes and behaviour.[118] In Scotland, the strategy for reducing the harm associated with alcohol use and misuse was set out by the SEHD in *Plan for action on alcohol problems* (SEHD, 2002).[120] This plan outlined the national communications strategy that incorporated a sustained mix of national and local activities spread over a period of years. In February 2007 the Scottish Executive published *Plan for action on alcohol problems: update* which provides an update on the original 2002 strategy.[80] This is very much focussed on issues wider than just health and outlines aims to change the culture of excessive drinking in Scotland as well as identifying progress on the previous plan and outlining aims for the future. The UK health departments also work with the Portman Group which has run a number of campaigns and initiatives to promote responsible drinking, reduce alcohol misuse and encourage responsible marketing.[121]

In England and Wales, alcohol education is a statutory requirement of the National Curriculum Science Order 1991, and schools are expected to use the non-statutory framework for personal, social and health education (PSHE) as the basis for extending their provision in this area. Alcohol education also features as one of the 10 themes of the National Healthy School Standard (NHSS). In Scotland, alcohol education is included in the ages 5-14 Health Education National Guidelines and NHS Health Scotland distributes teaching resources to schools, *Drink talking* and *Alcohol: what every parent should know*, that contain information on the effects of alcohol on the body and the health of unborn children. The current statutory curricular arrangements in Northern Ireland include a cross-curricular health education programme for young people aged between four and 16 years. Specifically, alcohol education is included within the Programmes of Study for Science and Technology (Key Stages 2-4).

In the UK, alcohol is relatively highly taxed compared to other European countries; however, the level of taxation is declining in real terms as the duty on spirits has not increased since 1997, and the duties on wine and beer have only increased in line with inflation.[122] In England and Wales, the Licensing Act 2003 permits a system of flexible opening hours for licensed premises, with the potential for up to 24-hour opening. The licensing systems in Scotland and Northern Ireland currently prohibit 24-hour opening.[m]

---

[m] In Scotland, the licensing system is regulated by the Licensing (Scotland) Act 1976, which prohibits 24-hour opening. However, as a result of regular extensions to licensing hours since 1976, Scotland has seen considerable liberalisation of opening hours. Under the Licensing Act 2005, a new system of licensing will come into force in Scotland in 2007 that includes a statutory presumption against 24-hour opening.

Appendix 5: T-ACE and TWEAK alcohol screening questionnaires

T-ACE

The T-ACE alcohol screening questionnaire consists of four questions that take less than a minute to answer:

1. Tolerance (T) – how many drinks does it take to make you feel high?
2. Annoyance (A) – have people annoyed you by criticising your drinking?
3. Cut down (C) – have you ever felt you ought to cut down on your drinking?
4. Eye-opener (E) – have you ever had a drink first thing in the morning to steady your nerves or get rid of a hangover?

A single point is given for an affirmative answer to the A, C and E questions, and two points are given when a pregnant woman indicates a tolerance of more than two drinks to feel high. A total score of two or more on the T-ACE test is suggestive of harmful drinking patterns during pregnancy.

Source: Sokol RJ, Martier SS & Ager JW (1989) The T-ACE questions: practical prenatal detection of risk-drinking. *American Journal of Obstetrics and Gynecology* **160**: 863-8.

TWEAK

There are two versions of the TWEAK screening questionnaire: one that is recommended for populations with high levels of binge drinking and one that is recommended for populations with low levels of binge drinking. Please note that as these questionnaires have been developed in the USA, the drinking levels stated refer to the USA levels.

The TWEAK alcohol screening questionnaire for populations with high levels of binge drinking consists of five questions:

1. Tolerance (T) – how many drinks does it take before the alcohol makes you fall asleep or pass out?
   Record number of drinks_____ (a positive score is six or more drinks)
   Or
   If you never drink until you pass out, what is the largest number of drinks that you have?
   Record number of drinks_____ (a positive score is six or more drinks)
2. Worried (W) – have your friends or relatives worried or complained about your drinking in the past year?
3. Eye opener (E) – do you sometimes take a drink in the morning when you first get up?
4. Amnesia (A) – are there times when you drink and you can't remember what you said or did?
5. Cut down (K) – do you sometimes feel the need to cut down on your drinking?

The TWEAK alcohol screening questionnaire for populations with low levels of binge drinking consists of five questions:

1. Tolerance (T) – how many drinks does it take before you begin to feel the first effects of alcohol?
   Record number of drinks_____ (a positive score is three or more drinks)
2. Worried (W) – have your friends or relatives worried or complained about your drinking in the past year?
3. Eye opener (E) – do you sometimes take a drink in the morning when you first get up?
4. Amnesia (A) – are there times when you drink and you can't remember what you said or did?
5. Cut down (K) – do you sometimes feel the need to cut down on your drinking?

For each version, a positive response to question T or W yields two points each, and an affirmative reply to question E, A or K scores one point each. A total score of two or more points on the TWEAK test is suggestive of harmful drinking patterns during pregnancy.

Source: Chan AWK, Pristach EA, Welte JW et al (1993) Use of the TWEAK test in screening for alcoholism/heavy drinking in three populations. *Alcoholism: Clinical and Experimental Research* **17**: 1188-92.

Appendix 6: indicated prevention interventions in the USA

A number of studies have assessed approaches aimed at preventing prenatal alcohol exposure in high-risk women. One of these approaches was the 'Protecting the next pregnancy' project. This project targets women who drank at risk levels during a previous pregnancy, and provides them with intensive brief intervention following the birth of a child affected by prenatal alcohol exposure. In comparison to a control group, the use of intensive brief interventions was found to reduce alcohol consumption during further pregnancies and subsequently resulted in improved birth outcomes.[75] A second approach, Project TrEAT (Trial for Early Alcohol Treatment), provided brief interventions for women between the ages of 18 and 40 who were identified as problem drinkers. Compared to a control group, women who received brief interventions were found to have reduced their mean alcohol intake and level of binge drinking, and to have reduced alcohol consumption during subsequent pregnancies.[75]

Appendix 7a: IoM diagnostic criteria for FASD

1. FAS with confirmed maternal alcohol exposure
A Confirmed maternal alcohol exposure
B Evidence of a characteristic pattern of facial anomalies that includes features such as short palpebral fissures and abnormalities in the premaxillary zone (eg flat upper lip, flattened philtrum, and flat midface)
C Evidence of growth retardation, as in at least one of the following:
  • low birth weight for gestational age
  • decelerating weight over time not due to nutrition
  • disproportional low weight to height.
D Evidence of CNS neurodevelopmental abnormalities, as in at least one of the following:
  • decreased cranial size at birth
  • structural brain abnormalities (eg microcephaly, partial or complete agenesis of the corpus callosum, cerebellar hypoplasia)
  • neurological hard or soft signs (as age appropriate), such as impaired fine motor skills, neurosensory hearing loss, poor tandem gait, poor eye-hand coordination.

2. FAS without confirmed maternal alcohol exposure
B, C, and D as above.

3. Partial FAS with confirmed maternal alcohol exposure
A Confirmed maternal alcohol exposure
B Evidence of some components of the pattern of characteristic facial anomalies
   Either C or D or E
C Evidence of growth retardation, as in at least one of the following:
  • low birth weight for gestational age
  • decelerating weight over time not due to nutrition
  • disproportional low weight to height.
D Evidence of CNS neurodevelopmental abnormalities, as in:
  • decreased cranial size at birth
  • structural brain abnormalities (eg microcephaly, partial or complete agenesis of the corpus callosum, cerebellar hypoplasia)
  • neurological hard or soft signs (as age appropriate) such as impaired fine motor skills, neurosensory hearing loss, poor tandem gait, poor eye hand coordination.
E Evidence of a complex pattern of behaviour or cognitive abnormalities that are inconsistent with developmental level and cannot be explained by familial background or environment alone, such as learning difficulties; deficits in school performance; poor impulse control; problems in social perception; deficits in higher level receptive and expressive language; poor capacity for abstraction or metacognition; specific deficits in mathematical skills; or problems in memory, attention, or judgment.

4. Alcohol-related birth defects (ARBD)

List of congenital anomalies, including malformations and dysplasias

Cardiac	Atrial septal defects	Aberrant great vessels	Ventricular septal defects	Tetralogy of Fallot
Skeletal	Hypoplastic nails	Clinodactyly	Shortened fifth digits	Pectus excavatum and carinatum
	Radioulnar synostosis Camptodactyly	Klippel-Feil syndrome Scoliosis	Flexion contractures	Hemivertebrae
Renal	Aplastic, dysplastic, Horseshoe kidneys	Ureteral duplications	Hypoplastic kidneys	Hydronephrosis
Ocular	Strabismus	Refractive problems secondary to small globes		Retinal vascular anomalies
Auditory	Conductive hearing loss	Neurosensory hearing loss		
Other	Virtually every malformation has been described in some patient with FAS. The etiologic specificity of most of these anomalies to alcohol teratogenesis remains uncertain.			

5. Alcohol-related neurodevelopmental disorder (ARND)

Presence of:

A   Evidence of CNS neurodevelopmental abnormalities, as in any one of the following:

- decreased cranial size at birth
- structural brain abnormalities (eg, microcephaly, partial or complete agenesis of the corpus callosum, cerebellar hypoplasia)
- neurological hard or soft signs (as age appropriate), such as impaired fine motor skills, neurosensory hearing loss, poor tandem gait, poor eye-hand coordination

and/or:

B   Evidence of a complex pattern of behavior or cognitive abnormalities that are inconsistent with developmental level and cannot be explained by familial background or environment alone, such as learning difficulties; deficits in school performance; poor impulse control; problems in social perception; deficits in higher level receptive and expressive language; poor capacity for abstraction or metacognition; specific deficits in mathematical skills; or problems in memory, attention, or judgment.

Source: Stratton KR, Howe CJ & Battaglia FC (1996) *Fetal alcohol syndrome: diagnosis, epidemiology, prevention and treatment.* Washington DC: National Academy Press.

Appendix 7b: proposed revised IoM criteria for FASD diagnosis

I. FAS With Confirmed Maternal Alcohol Exposure

(requires all features A–D)

A   Confirmed maternal alcohol exposure

B   Evidence of a characteristic pattern of minor facial anomalies, including   2 of the following:
1   short palpebral fissures (10th percentile)
2   thin vermilion border of the upper lip (score 4 or 5 with the lip/philtrum guide)
3   smooth philtrum (score 4 or 5 with the lip/philtrum guide)

C   Evidence of prenatal and/or postnatal growth retardation:
1   height or weight   10th percentile, corrected for racial norms, if possible

D   Evidence of deficient brain growth or abnormal morphogenesis, including   1 of the following:
1   structural brain abnormalities
2   head circumference   10th percentile

II. FAS Without Confirmed Maternal Alcohol Exposure

IB, IC, and ID, as above

III. Partial FAS With Confirmed Maternal Alcohol Exposure

(requires all features, A–C)

A   Confirmed maternal alcohol exposure

B   Evidence of a characteristic pattern of minor facial anomalies, including   2 of the following:
1   short palpebral fissures (10th percentile)
2   thin vermilion border of the upper lip (score 4 or 5 with the lip/philtrum guide)
3   smooth philtrum (score 4 or 5 with the lip/philtrum guide)

C   One of the following other characteristics:
1   evidence of prenatal and/or postnatal growth retardation:
a   height or weight   10th percentile corrected for racial norms, if possible
2   evidence of deficient brain growth or abnormal morphogenesis, including   1 of the following:
a   structural brain abnormalities
b   head circumference   10th percentile
3   evidence of a complex pattern of behavioural or cognitive abnormalities inconsistent with developmental level that cannot be explained by genetic predisposition, family background, or environment alone:
a   this pattern includes marked impairment in the performance of complex tasks (complex problem solving, planning, judgment, abstraction, metacognition, and arithmetic tasks); higher-level receptive and expressive language deficits; and disordered behaviour (difficulties in personal manner, emotional lability, motor dysfunction, poor academic performance, and deficient social interaction).

IV. Partial FAS Without Confirmed Maternal Alcohol Exposure

IIIB and IIIC, as above

V. ARBD (requires all features, A–C)

A Confirmed maternal alcohol exposure

B Evidence of a characteristic pattern of minor facial anomalies, including 2 of the following:

    1 short palpebral fissures (10th percentile)

    2 thin vermilion border of the upper lip (score 4 or 5 with the lip/philtrum guide)

    3 smooth philtrum (score 4 or 5 with the lip/philtrum guide)

C Congenital structural defects in 1 of the following categories, including malformations and dysplasias (if the patient displays minor anomalies only, 2 must be present): *cardiac*: atrial septal defects, aberrant great vessels, ventricular septal defects, conotruncal heart defects; *skeletal*: radioulnar synostosis, vertebral segmentation defects, large joint contractures, scoliosis; *renal*: aplastic/hypoplastic/dysplastic kidneys, 'horseshoe' kidneys/ureteral duplications; *eyes*: strabismus, ptosis, retinal vascular anomalies, optic nerve hypoplasia; *ears*: conductive hearing loss, neurosensory hearing loss; *minor anomalies*: hypoplastic nails, short fifth digits, clinodactyly of fifth fingers, pectus carinatum/excavatum, camptodactyly, 'hockey stick' palmar creases, refractive errors, 'railroad track' ears

VI. ARND (requires both A and B)

A Confirmed maternal alcohol exposure

B At least one of the following:

    1 evidence of deficient brain growth or abnormal morphogenesis, including 1 of the following:

        a structural brain abnormalities

        b head circumference 10th percentile

    2 evidence of a complex pattern of behavioral or cognitive abnormalities inconsistent with developmental level that cannot be explained by genetic predisposition, family background, or environment alone:

        a this pattern includes marked impairment in the performance of complex tasks (complex problem solving, planning, judgment, abstraction, metacognition, and arithmetic tasks); higher-level receptive and expressive language deficits; and disordered behaviour (difficulties in personal manner, emotional lability, motor dysfunction, poor academic performance, and deficient social interaction).

Source: Hoyme HU, May PA, Kalberg WO et al (2005) A practical clinical approach to diagnosis of fetal alcohol spectrum disorders: clarification of the 1996 Institute of Medicine Criteria. *Pediatrics* **115**: 39-47.

Appendix 8: CDC diagnostic criteria for FASD

Facial dysmorphia
Based on racial norms, individual exhibits all three characteristic facial features:
- smooth philtrum (University of Washington Lip-Philtrum Guide rank 4 or 5)
- thin vermillion border (University of Washington Lip-Philtrum Guide rank 4 or 5)
- small palpebral fissures (at or below 10th percentile).

Growth problems
Confirmed prenatal or postnatal height or weight, or both, at or below the 10th percentile, documented at any one point in time (adjusted for age, sex, gestational age, and race or ethnicity).

Central Nervous System Abnormalities
1   *Structural*
- Head circumference (OFC) at or below the 10th percentile adjusted for age and sex.
- Clinically significant brain abnormalities observable through imaging.
2   *Neurological*
Neurological problems not due to a postnatal insult or fever, or other soft neurological signs outside normal limits.
3   *Functional*
Performance substantially below that expected for an individual's age, schooling, or circumstances, as evidenced by:
- global cognitive or intellectual deficits representing multiple domains of deficit (or significant developmental delay in younger children) with performance below the 3rd percentile (2 standard deviations below the mean for standardised testing), or functional deficits below the 16th percentile (1 standard deviation below the mean for standardised testing) in at least three of the following domains:
  - a   cognitive or developmental deficits or discrepancies
  - b   executive functioning deficits
  - c   motor functioning delays
  - d   problems with attention or hyperactivity
  - e   social skills
  - f   other, such as sensory problems, pragmatic language problems, memory deficits, etc.

Maternal Alcohol Exposure
1   Confirmed prenatal alcohol exposure
2   Unknown prenatal alcohol exposure

Criteria for FAS Diagnosis
Requires all three of the following findings:
1   documentation of all three facial abnormalities (smooth philtrum, thin vermillion border, and small palpebral fissures);
2   documentation of growth deficits
3   documentation of CNS abnormality

Source: Bertrand J, Floyd RL, Weber MK et al (2005) *National task force on FAS/FAE: Guidelines for referral and diagnosis.* Atlanta: Centers for Disease Control and Prevention.

Appendix 9: 4-Digit diagnostic code

			3	4	4		4		
Severe	Severe	Definite (4)		X	X		X	(4)	High risk
			X						
Moderate	Moderate	Probable (3)						(3)	Some risk
Mild	Mild	Possible (2)						(2)	Unknown
None	None	Unlikely (1)	(1)	No risk					
Growth deficiency	**FAS facial features**	**CNS damage**	Growth	Face	CNS		Alcohol	**Prenatal alcohol**	

Source: Astley SJ (2006) Comparison of the 4-Digit code and the Hoyme diagnostic guidelines for Fetal Alcohol Spectrum Disorders. *Pediatrics* **118**: 1532-45.

The four digits of the diagnostic code reflect the magnitude of expression of the four key diagnostic features of FASD, in the following order: (1) growth deficiency, (2) FAS facial phenotype, (3) CNS abnormalities, and (4) prenatal alcohol exposure. There are 256 possible 4-digit diagnostic codes, ranging from 1111 to 4444. Each of the 4-digit diagnostic codes falls into one of 22 unique clinical diagnostic categories. Eight of the 22 diagnostic categories fall broadly under the designation of FASD. The 4-digit code (3444) that is inserted in the grid is one of the codes that meet the diagnostic criteria for FAS.

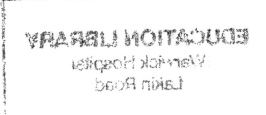

Appendix 10: Canadian FASD guidelines

The criteria for the diagnosis of fetal alcohol syndrome, after excluding other diagnoses, are:

A evidence of prenatal or postnatal growth impairment, as in at least one the following:

    a birth weight or birth length at or below the 10th percentile for gestational age.

    b height or weight at or below the 10th percentile for age.

    c disproportionately low weight-to-height ratio (= 10th percentile).

B simultaneous presentation of all three of the following facial anomalies at any age:

    a short palpebral fissure length (2 or more standard deviations below the mean).

    b smooth or flattened philtrum (rank 4 or 5 on the lip-philtrum guide).

    c thin upper lip (rank 4 or 5 on the lip-philtrum guide).

C evidence of impairment in three or more of the following CNS domains: hard and soft neurologic signs; brain structure; cognition; communication; academic achievement; memory; executive functioning and abstract reasoning; attention deficit/hyperactivity; adaptive behaviour, social skills, social communication.

D confirmed (or unconfirmed) maternal alcohol exposure.

The diagnostic criteria for partial fetal alcohol syndrome, after excluding other diagnoses, are:

A simultaneous presentation of two of the following facial anomalies at any age:

    a short palpebral fissure length (2 or more standard deviations below the mean).

    b smooth or flattened philtrum (rank 4 or 5 on the lip-philtrum guide).

    c thin upper lip (rank 4 or 5 on the lip-philtrum guide).

B evidence of impairment in three or more of the following central nervous system domains: hard and soft neurologic signs; brain structure; cognition; communication; academic achievement; memory; executive functioning and abstract reasoning; attention deficit/hyperactivity; adaptive behaviour, social skills, social communication.

C confirmed maternal alcohol exposure.

The diagnostic criteria for alcohol-related neurodevelopmental disorder, after excluding other diagnoses, are:

A evidence of impairment in three or more of the following CNS domains: hard and soft neurologic signs; brain structure; cognition; communication; academic achievement; memory; executive functioning and abstract reasoning; attention deficit/hyperactivity; adaptive behaviour, social skills, social communication.

B confirmed maternal alcohol exposure.

The term alcohol-related birth defects (ARBD) should not be used as an umbrella or diagnostic term, for the spectrum of alcohol effects. ARBD constitutes a list of congenital anomalies, including malformations and dysplasias and should be used with caution

Source: Chudley AE, Conry J, Cook JL et al (2005) Fetal alcohol spectrum disorder: Canadian guidelines for diagnosis. *Can Med Assoc J* **172**: s1–s21.

References

1   British Medical Association (2005) *Binge drinking*. London: British Medical Association.

2   Mukherjee RAS, Hollnis S & Turk J (2006) Fetal alcohol spectrum disorder: an overview. *Journal of the Royal Society of Medicine* **99**: 298-302.

3   Lupton C, Burd L & Harwood R (2004) Cost of fetal alcohol spectrum disorders. *American Journal of Medical Genetics* **127C**: 42-50.

4   Gray R & Henderson J (2006) *Review of the fetal effects of prenatal alcohol exposure. Report to the Department of Health*. Oxford: National Perinatal Epidemiology Unit, University of Oxford.

5   Welch-Carre E (2005) The neurodevelopmental consequences of prenatal alcohol exposure. *Advances in Neonatal Care* **5**: 217-29.

6   Williamson J, Sham P & Ball D (2003) Binge drinking trends in a UK community-based sample. *Journal of Substance Use* **8**: 234-7.

7   Plant MA, Miller P & Plant ML (2005) Trends in drinking, smoking and illicit drug use among 15 and 16 year olds in the United Kingdom (1995-2003). *Journal of Substance Use*. **10**: 331-9.

8   Plant MA & Plant ML (2006) *Binge Britain: alcohol and the national response*. Oxford: Oxford University Press.

9   Sokol RJ, Delaney-Black V & Nordstrom B (2003) Fetal alcohol spectrum disorder. *Journal of the American Medical Association* **290**: 2996-9.

10   Murphy-Brennan MG & Oei TPS (1999) Is there evidence to show that fetal alcohol syndrome can be prevented. *Journal of Drug Education* **29**: 5-24.

11   Department of Health Hospital Episode Statistics (HES) 2002-03.

12   NHS National Services Scotland (2006) Data provided by the Substance Misuse Team, ISD Scotland.

13   May PA and Gossage JP (2001) Estimating the prevalence of fetal alcohol syndrome – a summary. *Alcohol and Health Research* **25**: 159-67.

14   Abel EL (1998) Fetal alcohol syndrome: the 'American Paradox'. *Alcohol & Alcoholism* **333**: 195-201.

15   Abel EL & Sokel RJ (1987) Incidence of fetal alcohol syndrome and economic impact of FAS-related anomalies. *Drug and Alcohol Dependence* **19**: 51-70.

16   Hancock R (2004) Prevalence of fetal alcohol syndrome in a remote region of Australia. *Journal of FAS International* **2**: e5.

17   Maya PA, Gossage PJ, Marais AS et al (In press) The epidemiology of fetal alcohol syndrome and partial FAS in a South African community. *Drug and Alcohol Dependence*.

18   May PA, Fiorentino, DJ, Gossage P et al (2006) Epidemiology of FASD in a province in Italy: prevalence and characteristics of children in a random sample of schools. *Alcoholism: Clinical and Experimental Research* **30**: 1562-75.

19   Stade BC, Stevens B, Ungar WJ et al (2006) Health-related quality of life of Canadian children and youth prenataly exposed to alcohol. *Health & Quality of Life Outcomes* **4**: 81.

20   Autti-Rämö I (2002) Foetal alcohol syndrome – a multifaceted condition. *Developmental Medicine and Child Neurology* **44**: 141-4.

21   Bertrand J, Floyd RL, Weber MK et al (2005) *National task force on FAS/FAE. Fetal alcohol syndrome: guidelines for referral and diagnosis*. Atlanta: Centers for Disease Control and Prevention.

22   Plant ML (1997) *Women and alcohol: contemporary and historical perspectives*. London: Free Association Books.

23   Academy of Medical Sciences (2004) *Calling time: the nation's drinking as a health issue*. London: Academy of Medical Sciences.

24   Cabinet Office Prime Minister's Strategy Unit (2004) *Alcohol harm reduction strategy for England*. London: Cabinet Office.

25   Plant ML & Plant MA (2001) Heavy drinking by young British women gives cause for concern. *British Medical Journal* **323**: 1183.

26   Plant ML, Plant MA & Mason W (2002) Drinking, smoking and illicit drug use amongst British adults: gender differences explored. *Journal of Substance Use* **7**: 24-33.

27   Office for National Statistics (2005) *Results from the 2003 General Household Survey*. London: Her Majesty's Stationery Office.

28   Parliamentary Office of Science and Technology (2005) *Binge drinking and public health*. London: The Parliamentary Office of Science and Technology.

29   Office for National Statistics (2006) *National Statistics Omnibus Survey*. London: Her Majesty's Stationery Office.

30   Department of Health (2001) *Annual report of the Chief Medical Officer*. London: Department of Health.

31   Hamlyn B, Brooker S, Oleinikova K et al (2002) *Infant feeding survey 2000. National Health Service Information Centre*. London: Her Majesty's Stationery Office.

32   British Medical Association (2003) *Adolescent health*. London: British Medical Association.

33   Health Development Agency (2004) *Teenage pregnancy: an overview of the research evidence*. London: Health Development Agency.

34   Office for National Statistics (2007) *Health Statistics Quarterly 33*. London: Her Majesty's Stationery Office.

35   NHS National Services Scotland (2005) *Teenage pregnancy*. Edinburgh: NHS National Services Scotland.

36   Family Planning Association Northern Ireland (2003) *Teenage pregnancy*. Belfast: Family Planning Association Northern Ireland.

37   The UK Collaborative Group for HIV and STI Surveillance (2006) *A complex picture. HIV and other sexually transmitted infections in the United Kingdom: 2006*. London: Health Protection Agency, Centre for Infections.

38   Dex S & Joshi H (ed) (2005) *Children of the 21st century: from birth to nine months*. Bristol: Policy Press.

39   Lakha F & Glasier A (2006) Unintended pregnancy and use of emergency contraception among a large cohort of women attending for antenatal care or abortion in Scotland. *Lancet* **368**: 1782-7.

40   Sherman CA, Harvey SM & Noell J (2005) 'Are they still having sex?' STI's and unintended pregnancy among mid-life women. *Journal of Women & Aging* **17**: 41-55.

41   Riley EP & McGee CL (2005) Fetal alcohol spectrum disorders: an overview with emphasis on changes in brain and behaviour. *Experimental Biology and Medicine* **230**: 357-65.

42   Plant ML, Abel EL & Guerri C (1999) Alcohol and Pregnancy. In: I Macdonald (ed) *Health issues related to alcohol consumption*. Oxford: Blackwell Science.

43   Abel EL (2006) Fetal alcohol syndrome: a cautionary note. *Current Pharmaceutical Design* **12**: 1521-9.

44   O'Leary CM (2004) Fetal alcohol syndrome: diagnosis, epidemiology, and developmental outcomes. *Journal of Paediatrics and Child Health* **40**: 2-7.

45   Warren KR & Ting-Kai LI (2005) Genetic polymorphisms: Impact on the risk of fetal alcohol spectrum disorders. *Birth Defects Research* **73**: 195-203.

46   Kotch LE & Sulik KK (1992) Experimental fetal alcohol syndrome: proposed pathogenic basis for a variety of associated facial and brain anomalies. *American Journal of Medical Genetics* **44**: 168-76.

47   Chen S, Periasamy A, Yang B et al (2000) Differential sensitivity of mouse neural crest cells to ethanol-induced toxicity. *Alcohol* **20**: 75-81.

48   Dunty WC, Chen S, Zucker RM et al (2001) Selective vulnerability of embryonic cell populations to ethanol-induced apoptosis: implications for alcohol-related birth defects and neurodevelopmental disorder. *Alcoholism: Clinical and Experimental Research* **25**: 1523-35.

49   Sulik KK (2005) Genesis of alcohol-induced craniofacial dysmorphism. *Experimental Biology and Medicine* **230**: 366-75.

50   Autti-Rämö I, Autti T, Korkman M et al (2002) MRI findings in children with school problems who had been exposed prenatally to alcohol. *Developmental Medicine & Child Neurology* **44**: 98-106.

51   Royal College of Obstetricians and Gynaecologists (2006) *Alcohol consumption and the outcomes of pregnancy*. London: Royal College of Obstetricians and Gynaecologists.

52   Ikonomidou C, Bittigau P, Ishimaru MJ et al (2000) Ethanol-induced apoptotic neurodegeneration and fetal alcohol syndrome. *Science* **287**: 1056-60.

53   Mukherjee RAS, Hollins S, Abou-Saleh MT et al (2005) Low level alcohol consumption and the fetus. *British Medical Journal* **330**: 375-6.

54   Sood B, Delaney-Black V, Covington C et al (2001) Prenatal alcohol exposure and childhood behavior at Age 6 to 7 Years: I. Dose-response effect. *Pediatrics* **108**: e34 (electronic article).

55   Akay M & Mulder EJH (1996) Investigating the effect of maternal alcohol intake on human fetal breathing rate using adaptive time-frequency analysis methods. *Early Human Development* **46**: 153-64.

56   McLeod W, Brien JF, Loomis C et al (1983) Effects of maternal ethanol ingestion on fetal breathing movements gross body movements and heart rate at 37 to 40 weeks gestational age. *American Journal of Obstetrics and Gynaecology* **145**: 251-7.

57   Fox HE, Steinbrecher M & Pessel D (1978) Maternal ethanol ingestion and the occurrence of human fetal breathing movements. *American Journal of Obstetrics and Gynecology* **132**: 354-8.

58   Mulder EJH, Morssink LP & van der Schee (1998) Acute maternal alcohol consumption disrupts behavioral state organization in the near-term fetus. *Pediatric Research* **44**: 774-9.

59   Little JF, Hepper PG & Dornan JC (2002) Maternal alcohol consumption during pregnancy and fetal startle behaviour. *Physiology and Behavior* **76**: 691-4.

60   Hepper PG, Dornan JC & Little JF (2005) Maternal alcohol consumption during pregnancy may delay the development of spontaneous fetal startle behaviour. *Physiology and Behavior* **83**: 711-4.

61   Sayal K, Heron J & Golding J (2007) Prenatal alcohol exposure and gender differences in childhood mental health problems: a longitudinal population-based study. *Paediatrics* **119**: 426-34.

62   Goodlett CR & Horn KH (2001) Mechanisms of alcohol-induced damage to the developing nervous system. *Alcohol Research & Health* **25**: 175-84.

63   Goodlett CR, Horn KH & Zhou FC (2005) Alcohol teratogenesis: mechanisms of damage and strategies for intervention. *Experimental Biology & Medicine* **230**: 394-406.

64   Hepper PG (1992) Fetal psychology. An embryonic science. In: Nijhuis, JG (ed) (1992) *Fetal behaviour. Developmental and perinatal aspects.* Oxford: Oxford University Press.

65   Jensen TK, Hjollund NHI, Henriksen TB et al (1998) Does moderate alcohol consumption affect fertility? Follow up study among couples planning first pregnancy. *British Medical Journal* **317**: 505-10.

66   Kesmodel U, Wisborg K & Olsen SF (2002) Moderate alcohol intake during pregnancy and the risk of stillbirth and death in the first year of life. *American Journal of Epidemiology* **155**: 305-12.

67   www.nichd.nih.gov/research/supported/pass.cfm

68   Mukherjee RAS, Hollnis S & Turk J (2006) Psychiatric comorbidity in foetal alcohol syndrome. *Psychiatric Bulletin* **30**: 194-5.

69   Elliott EJ, Payne J, Haan E et al (2006) Diagnosis of foetal alcohol syndrome and alcohol use in pregnancy: a survey of paediatricians' knowledge, attitudes and practice. *Journal of Paediatrics and Child Health* **42**: 698-703.

70   Gahagan S, Sharpe TT, Brimacombe M et al (2006) Paediatrician's knowledge, training, and experience in the care of children with fetal alcohol syndrome. *Pediatrics* **118**: e657-68.

71   Payne J, Elliot E, D'Antoine H et al (2005) Health professionals' knowledge, practice and opinions about fetal alcohol syndrome and alcohol consumption in pregnancy. *Australia and New Zealand Journal of Public Health* **29**: 558-64.

72   Nevin AC, Parshuram C & Nulman I (2002) A survey of physicians knowledge regarding awareness of maternal alcohol use and the diagnosis of FAS. *BMC Family Practice* **3**: 2.

73   Diekman ST, Floyd RL & Decoufle P (2000) A survey of obstetrician-gynecologists on their patients' alcohol use during pregnancy. *Obstetrics and Gynecology* **95**: 756-63.

74   United States Department of Health and Human Services press release (21.02.05) *US Surgeon General Releases Advisory on Alcohol Use in Pregnancy.*

75   Hankin JR (2002) Fetal alcohol syndrome prevention research. *Alcohol Research and Health* **26**: 58-65.

76   Abel EL (1998) Prevention of alcohol abuse-related birth effects – I. Public education efforts. *Alcohol and Alcoholism* **33**: 411-6.

77   Eustace LW, Kang DH & Coombs D (2003) Fetal alcohol syndrome: a growing concern for health care professionals. *Journal of Obstetric, Gynecologic and Neonatal Nursing* **32**: 215-21.

78   Armstrong EM & Abel EL (2000) Fetal alcohol syndrome: the origins of a moral panic. *Alcohol and Alcoholism* **35**: 276-82.

79   Room R, Babor T & Rehm J (2005) Alcohol and public health. *Lancet* **365**: 519-30.

80   Scottish Executive Health Department (2007) *Plan for action on alcohol problems: update*. Edinburgh: Scottish Executive Health Department.

81   Abel EL (1998) Prevention of alcohol abuse-related birth effects – II. Targeting and pricing. *Alcohol and Alcoholism* **33**: 417-20.

82   Mukherjee RAS (2006) Fetal alcohol spectrum disorders. *MIMMS* Women's health **1**: 28-30.

83   Chang G (2004) Screening and brief intervention in prenatal care settings. *Alcohol Research and Health* **28**: 80-4.

84   Bearer CF (2001) Markers to detecting drinking during pregnancy. *Alcohol Research and Health* **25**: 210-8.

85   Stoller JM & Holmes LB (1999) Under recognition of prenatal alcohol effects in infants of known alcohol abusing women. *Journal of Pediatrics* **135**: 430-6.

86   Littner Y & Bearer CF (2007) Detection of alcohol consumption during pregnancy – current and future biomarkers. *Neuroscience & Biobehavioral Reviews* **31**: 261-9.

87   Chan D, Caprara D, Blanchette P et al (2004) Recent developments in meconium and hair testing methods for the confirmation of gestational exposures to alcohol and tobacco smoke. *Clinical Biochemistry* **37**: 429-38.

88   Sokol RJ, Martier SS & Ager JW (1989) The T-ACE questions: practical detection of risk-drinking. *American Journal of Obstetrics and Gynecology* **160**: 863-70.

89   Chan AK, Pristach EA, Welte JW et al (1993) The TWEAK test in screening for alcoholism/heavy drinking in three populations. *Alcoholism: Clinical and Experimental Research* **6**: 1188-92.

90   Floyd RL, O'Connor MJ, Bertrand J et al (2006) Reducing adverse outcomes from prenatal alcohol exposure: a clinical plan of action. *Alcoholism: Clinical and Experimental Research* **30**: 1271-5.

91   Savage C, Wray J, Ritchey PN et al (2003) Current screening instruments related to alcohol consumption in pregnancy and a proposed alternative method. *Journal of Obstetric, Gynecologic, and Neonatal Nursing* **32**: 437-46.

92   National Treatment Agency for Substance Misuse (2006) *Review of the effectiveness for alcohol problems*. London: National Treatment Agency for Substance Misuse.

93   Scottish Executive Health Department (2004) *Effective and cost-effective measures to reduce alcohol misuse in Scotland: an update to the literature review*. Edinburgh: Scottish Executive Health Department.

94   Department of Health (2006) *Models of care for adult alcohol misusers*. London: Department of Health.

95   Scottish Intercollegiate Guidelines Network (2003) *The management of harmful drinking and alcohol dependence in primary care*. Edinburgh: Scottish Intercollegiate Guidelines Network.

96   Health Development Agency (2002) Manual for the fast alcohol screen test (FAST): fast screening for alcohol problems. London: Health Development Agency.

97   National Institute for Health and Clinical Excellence (2003) *Antenatal care: routine care for the healthy pregnant woman*. London: National Institute for Health and Clinical Excellence.

98   O'Connor MJ & Whaley SE (2007) Brief intervention for alcohol use by pregnant women. *American Journal of Public Health* **97**: 252-8.

99   Chang G, McNamara TK & Orav EJ (2005) Brief intervention for prenatal alcohol use: a randomized trial. *Obstetrics and Gynecology* **105**: 991-8.

100   Abel EL (1988) Fetal alcohol syndrome in families. *Neurotoxicology and Teratology* **10**: 1-2.

101   www.ncbi.nlm.nih.gov/books/bv.fcgi?rid=hstat5.chapter.22442 (accessed May 2007)

102   Floyd RL, O'Connor MJ, Sokol RJ et al (2005) Recognition and prevention of fetal alcohol syndrome. *Obstetrics and Gynecology* **106**: 1059-64.

103   Nevin AC, Parshuram C, Nulman I et al (2002) A survey of physicians knowledge regarding awareness of maternal alcohol use and the diagnosis of FAS. *BMC Family Practice* **3**: 2.

104   Jones KL (1997) *Smith's recognisable patterns of human malformations*. (5e) Philadelphia: WB Saunders and Co.

105   Centers for Disease Control and Prevention (2004) *Fetal alcohol syndrome: guidelines for referral and diagnosis*. Atlanta: Centers for Disease Control and Prevention.

106   Hoyme HU, May PA, Kalberg WO et al (2005) A practical clinical approach to diagnosis of fetal alcohol spectrum disorders: clarification of the 1996 Institute of Medicine Criteria. *Pediatrics* **115**: 39-47.

107   Astley SJ (2006) Comparison of the 4-digit diagnostic code and Hoyme diagnostic guidelines for fetal alcohol spectrum disorders. *Pediatrics* **118**: 1532-45.

108   National Institute for Health and Clinical Excellence (2003) *Antenatal care: routine care for the healthy pregnant woman. Information for pregnant women, their families and the public*. London: National Institute for Health and Clinical Excellence.

109   Department of Health (2006) *How much is too much? Pregnancy and alcohol*. London: Department of Health.

110   NHS Health Scotland (2003) *Alcofacts – a guide to sensible drinking*. Edinburgh: NHS Health Scotland.

111   Health Promotion Agency for Northern Ireland (2006) *Focus on alcohol – a guide to drinking and health*. Belfast: Health Promotion Agency for Northern Ireland.

112   Hepper PG (1995) The behaviour of the foetus as an indicator of neural functioning In: Lecanuet JP, Fifer WP, Krasnegor NA et al (eds) *Fetal development: A psychobiological perspective*. New Jersey: Lawrence Erlbaum.

113   Hata T, Kanenishi K, Akiyama M et al (2005) Real-time 3-D sonographic observation of fetal facial expression. *Journal of Obstetrics and Gynaecology Research* **31**: 337-40.

114   Kurjak A, Carrera JM, Stanojevic M et al (2005) The antenatal development of fetal behavioral patterns assessed by four-dimensional sonography. *The Journal of Maternal-Fetal and Neonatal Medicine* **17**: 401-16.

115   Mulder EJH, Kamstra A, O'Brien MJ et al (1986). Abnormal fetal behavioural state regulation in a case of high maternal alcohol intake during pregnancy. *Early Human Development* **14**: 321-326.

116   Castillo RA, Devoe LD, Ruedrich DA et al (1989). The effects of acute alcohol intoxication on biophysical activities: A case report. *American Journal of Obstetrics and Gynaecology.* **160**: 692-3

117   Department of Health (1995) *Sensible drinking*. London: Department of Health.

118   Prime Minister's Strategy Unit (2004) *Alcohol harm reduction strategy for England*. London: Prime Minister's Strategy Unit.

119   Department of Health (2004) *Choosing health: making healthier choices easier*. London: Department of Health.

120   Scottish Executive Health Department (2002) *Plan for action on alcohol problems*. Edinburgh: Scottish Executive Health Department.

121   www.portmangroup.org.uk

122   Institute of Alcohol Studies (2005) *Alcohol: tax, price and public health*. Cambridge: Institute of Alcohol Studies.

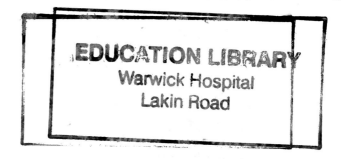